One in a Million
My Story

Steve Prescott MBE
With Mike Critchley and Linzi Prescott

Vertical Editions
www.verticaleditions.com

First published in the United Kingdom in 2014 by Vertical Editions, Unit 4a, Snaygill Industrial Estate, Skipton, North Yorkshire BD23 2QR

www.verticaleditions.com

ISBN 978-1-904091-84-4

A CIP catalogue record for this book is available from the British Library

Cover design by HBA, York

Manufacturing managed by Jellyfish Solutions Ltd, Swanmore
Printed and bound by Gutenberg Press Ltd, Malta

Linzi; you have been my rock. I don't know what I would have done without you by my side.

My beautiful boys; for bringing me so much happiness, and for your understanding when we had to be apart. I am so proud of you both.

Anil Vaidya and the transplant team at The Churchill Hospital, Oxford; thank you for your commitment, positivity, expertise and primarily for giving me hope! My family and I are indebted to you.

Steve Prescott MBE, October 2013

I'd like to thank everybody involved in Stephen's care, particularly Mark Saunders, Tom Cecil and Anil Vaidya. Also all the ambassadors and SPF members for continuing Stephen's work and to all our family and friends for the support they have given to me and the boys.

Linzi Prescott, July 2014

Contents

Part 2: Linzi Takes Up the Story

Part 3: Postscript by Mr Anil Vaidya, Consultant Transplant Surgeon from Oxford's Churchill Hospital

Acknowledgments

Stephen began writing his autobiography with the help of *St Helens Star* journalist Mike Critchley in September 2007 and the manuscript was more or less complete shortly before his passing in November 2013.

The book's initial script was very quickly overtaken by the way Stephen fought cancer and every year there was always another challenge, something bigger to write about and another major revision.

Stephen revised and refined six years worth of written content during his lengthy stay in hospital in 2013.

The book has been a long time in writing but thanks go to all those who have helped along the way. Saints historian Alex Service assisted in the writing of three of the early chapters and provided the statistics at the end. Thanks also to David Burke, who proof read the manuscript before publication, and to Bernard Platt and RLphotos.com for their excellent photographs.

Massive thanks also go to all those people who gave up their time to write such lovely, glowing tributes to Stephen.

Linzi Prescott

Foreword

Linzi Prescott

Pseudomyxoma peritonei, often referred to as PMP, is a condition which arises from a tumour on the appendix. When Stephen was diagnosed in 2006 he was told that it was so rare that it only affects one in a million.

That was the reason he chose those words as the title of his autobiography, however, now Stephen is no longer with us, the title means so much more to me.

Stephen really was one in a million and certainly not because of the hand he was dealt, but because of the person, husband and dad he was.

I have never met, nor will I ever meet, anyone as special as Stephen. I am incredibly proud of the extraordinary, positive and determined way in which he approached his life despite the odds. Being diagnosed with cancer changed our lives and moulded the person Stephen became.

He dedicated the last years of his life to his family and to helping others through the Steve Prescott Foundation.

With pseudomyxoma being so rare it doesn't get the funding for research like more common forms of the disease. This was one of the reasons behind the initial fundraising, seeing the formation of the charity. Stephen received so much help from the general public because of his rugby league profile and he was overwhelmed. He realised that not everybody is so lucky and he wanted to support others and give something back by helping people like him and in the process raise awareness of this dreadful disease.

Stephen knew that only a cure would help him and he never gave up the search. His single-mindedness led him to Oxford's Churchill Hospital for a ground-breaking, pioneering modified multivisceral transplant which would give him a new set of organs and remove the tumour, giving him a potential cure of this devastating condition and a second chance of life.

Unfortunately, despite the optimism immediately after the 32 hour operation, we did not get the successful outcome that everybody involved desperately hoped for.

On November 9, 2013 Stephen passed away after multiple organ failure caused by graft versus host disease – a complication following the transplant.

I take comfort in the fact that Stephen passed away so full of hope and positivity for the future, and the disease he had battled for so long had all gone. We knew that Stephen couldn't have survived without the transplant.

Nobody knows what we went through during the last seven years of Stephen's life, particularly the last eight months. However, the chance of the transplant offered us a lifeline which we never imagined possible. We knew the risks from the onset but they didn't concern Stephen. He wanted to beat the disease and he knew this was his only option. He got his dream. I have absolutely no regrets and if I could turn back time I would still make the same choices.

I feel very proud at Stephen's bravery in going through with this 'first in the world' surgery and lessons learned from the experience may help other patients with pseudomyxoma in the future.

With that, and the legacy of the Steve Prescott Foundation, his life will continue to help many, through the charities the SPF supports, all of which were very close to his heart – The Christie, Try Assist and now the Oxford Transplant Foundation.

Stephen will continue to inspire people to keep fighting and never give up. He certainly inspires me every day. He fought so hard to get extra time to spend with our boys and during those weeks, months and years he was able to instil in them the qualities and virtues that are truly important in life and they will continue his legacy. That, along with the renaming of the Man of Steel Award, means that his name will live on forever.

Part 1
Steve's Story

Introduction

Friday, September 8, 2006 should have been the happiest day of our lives. It certainly started that way with the tears of joy flowing freely in the early hours of the morning after my wife Linzi had given birth to little Koby Zak Stephen Prescott. Within hours, alas, the tears were those of fear, worry and pure devastation rolling down my cheeks after being given crushing news that would turn mine and my family's life completely upside down. The contrast, in just a matter of a few hours, could never have been starker.

I will never forget that morning – the sight of Linzi picking up Koby and saying, 'Aw, look at him, he's beautiful.' She was not wrong and I put Koby on my chest. He was perfect. When I went home a couple of hours later to tell Taylor he had a brother, I was so unbelievably happy that our family was now complete.

Later on in the afternoon all the neighbours came out to welcome Linzi and the new baby home from hospital and we had champagne, fun and jokes in the street. But the time passed quickly and I had to leave the celebration to head over for an appointment at the East Yorkshire BUPA hospital because I wanted to get to the bottom of the pains I had been experiencing in my abdomen.

Little did we know that a bombshell was about to be dropped on our perfect world. The truth is that the specialist did not need to say anything to me; I already knew something was badly wrong when I saw his face change after he had finished examining my stomach and abdomen. Then he delivered the crushing news that in all likelihood I had lymphoma and ordered me to go for CT scans and blood tests.

Cancer. The mere mention of the word absolutely petrified me and I burst into tears walking back to the car park. We hoped for the best, comforted ourselves with thoughts of a worst-case scenario, but alas it was true.

'Have you ever heard of metastatic cancer?' asked the nurse practitioner when Linzi and I returned to hospital for my test results a week later.

'It means you have tumours everywhere in your abdomen. It's inoperable and incurable.'

Her words made me numb, but I fired away with questions nonetheless. She interpreted the last one for me saying, 'If you are asking me if you're going to see your boys grow up then the answer is no.' It is just not possible to describe the emotion I went through when I was told I was going to die and not see my two boys grow up.

Those words ripped through me; like somebody had plunged a knife in my heart and ripped it out. I was devastated. We all were. All I was thinking at the time was that I had no hope, no life and I had nothing in my body to fight. They had put me in a dark tunnel with no sign of a light at the end of it.

We went over to St Helens that weekend where my close friends Mike Ford and Paul Barrow came round to see me to try to give me some motivation. For all that I hoped, prayed and wished I really needed a start line – but for the life of me I just could not see it.

Linzi rang some of our other friends to break the bad news before they heard it from somebody else, but I shut myself off in my room, unable to face the world. I just wanted to curl up and block everything out

One phone call changed that and as soon as Linzi told Steve Crooks, my old coach and friend, he was hammering at my front door. Crooksy came up to my room and made me go and sit downstairs. In his own straight-talking way he said, 'Steve, if you have got one day, one week or one month I know you will fight it.' That is what helped motivate me and was just what I needed to hear. Although I was a wreck, when he came in and gave me that talk it kind of picked me up. This was a real turning point in the way I was going to handle this – how I was going to face the world and fight cancer.

I was at the start line – and that is just where I needed to be after some really dark, bewildering days.

Further tests revealed I had a rare cancer called pseudomyxoma peritonei, one which affects one in a million people, a disease that tends to start in the appendix. Although we don't know how long I had it, it was explained that pseudomyxoma peritonei was a slow growing cancer. Also, instead of the few months I had initially been told I had to live, my prognosis was now three to five years. So, although there was still a dark outlook, we were elated that there was more hope.

And with hope came fight and, with Linzi always by my side, I made sure that I was going to hit this disease with every fibre of my being.

When you are told devastating news it can either go two ways, you can go downhill, or you can fight and go uphill. I decided to go uphill, get on with my life and try to enjoy being with my family the best way I could.

After I was first diagnosed with cancer I received loads of help from the rugby league community and general public, starting with forums, a gala dinner and a boxing event followed by a charity game involving some of my former team-mates at Knowsley Road.

That day in particular played a massive part in inspiring me to set about the gruelling challenges I went on to face later. It dawned on me I was not finished yet and I could do something myself to inspire other people. Yes, I was frail. I had lost a lot of weight having been through a major operation and having organs removed but it gives you such a lift when you realise people are willing to help you and you see thousands backing you. The rugby league community certainly showed me that day that they were going to be with me every step of the way for my battle against cancer.

I set up the Steve Prescott Foundation because of all the help I received – it made me want to help other people in return. My charity challenges were not only about raising money, but I also wanted to show other people with cancer that we can fight it, even beat it, and carry on living and enjoying our lives.

This is my story.

1

Growing Up in St Helens

It was first time around for Slade's number one 'Merry Xmas Everybody'. Noddy Holder's distinctive holler was ringing out when I came into the world four weeks early at home on Boxing Day 1973, weighing in at 6lb 4oz. With it being the feast of St Stephen there was probably only one name for me. Many happy days and years were spent at that loving family home in Wingate Avenue, in the Nutgrove area of St Helens – and my parents still live there today. I was brought up well with my brother Neil, who was not much older than me and our sister Suzanne who came along nine years later. My mum and dad were very supportive and although I followed in my dad's sporting footsteps I do get a lot of traits from my mum – I am stubborn, too.

When it came to sport, me and my older brother were very competitive and always had a ball – be it round or oval. Sport was in the blood, so to speak. My dad, who was a semi-professional rugby league player, encouraged me to play a full variety of sports. He bought me my first rugby ball, which I duly kicked through the kitchen window. He even bought me some golf clubs and so we used to nip up to the neighbouring Sherdley Park course to practise, invariably getting chased off by the park keeper. Our mini Wembley was the nearby Nutgrove Hall Drive field or the patch of land known locally as 'the Clegg' – a place where me and our Neil would vie to score the winning goal or try before getting called in for our tea. A competitive streak was always there within me and, without wishing to sound big headed, I always won races at sports days and local field days, especially the St Austin's church parish gala. Although I took my sport seriously, I never realised I had talent, it was something that came naturally to me. It wasn't just ball games and running – when I was a pupil at De La Salle, I broke the Merseyside schools high jump record and held it for over a decade. Years later a rugby fan wrote to me when I was playing for Hull FC and told me that they had just broken my record.

Away from school I combined playing rugby league at St Helens Crusaders junior outfit, now Thatto Heath, with football at local youth team Parr and Hardshaw. I doubled up for three years until I was 12 when it became too much for me. Well, that's what my parents told me. I have now learnt, through my own children, that it was probably too much for them really, with all the travelling that goes with it. It reached a point where my dad told me to make a decision on which sport to pursue, so I chose to concentrate on football.

As a youngster, I had some interest from the professional clubs' scouts and it felt great having trials at Tranmere Rovers and training at Wigan Athletic, even though they were lower league minnows at Springfield Park back then. Burnley also enquired, and on another occasion Liverpool scouts watched me play a big local derby for Parr and Hardshaw against Penlake. Unfortunately, I missed a penalty in that game and, not surprisingly, never heard anything from the Reds afterwards. However, I did eventually make it to Anfield – if only as a Parr and Hardshaw player! Our five-a-side team won an all-Merseyside competition and qualified for the finals at Liverpool's famous stadium for two years in a row. We lost both times in the final – and although I scored, we lost twice on penalties and I again missed one. It was a great experience though, particularly with me being a Liverpool fan.

Academically, I didn't really set the world on fire, getting a few Cs but a lot of D grades in my GCSEs, but I did okay at Business Studies and Art. The following year I went to Carmel College and got a B in Sports Science, which probably showed where my interests lay.

My school reports at Edmund Campion and then De La Salle were not bad, but I never revised or concentrated much because I was always training. Although I liked History and Art, I absolutely loved sport. It used to infuriate my mum because every time she went to parents' evenings at school, the teachers would tell her how good I was at football and rugby, but all she wanted to know was how good I was at English and Maths. She wanted me to be a teacher or have a trade to fall back on, rather than relying on my sporting pipe-dreams being fulfilled. I didn't have a set career path – it was simply a case of it developing as the years went by.

If truth be known sport was the main thing I got from my hours, days and weeks at school. Although I played for the school teams, every dinner break you would find me with a ball at my feet. I played the lot – football, rugby union, a little bit of rugby league and cricket.

In the third year at De La Salle, when I was aged 14, I broke my ankle which meant me having a bit of time off school. No sooner was the plaster taken off I started with severe stomach pains. After struggling in agony for nearly a week, my dad took me to the doctor who diagnosed an abscess on my appendix and sent me to hospital. They could not take the abscess out there and then but drained it and, despite all that I have been through since, I can still picture the big rubber gas mask being placed on my face. The whole hideous experience gave me a fear of needles, too. A few weeks later, when I had to go in to hospital again to finally have the appendix out, I was so terrified that my mum had to bribe me with a new Berghaus jacket before I would leave the house. I don't know the fine details but when they operated they left the stump of my appendix attached. If they hadn't left it in it would not have been possible to be struck with pseudomyxoma peritonei because that disease has its origin on the appendix. That was such a small detail and yet it has had quite a massive consequence on my life.

On leaving school at 16, I went on to Carmel Sixth Form College to re-sit some GCSEs and pick up Sports. After a year I realised that college wasn't for me and I took an apprenticeship-type course at Stoves, which was a massive oven factory in Rainhill, on the outskirts of St Helens. There I learned to weld and use drills and lathes. Punctuality was a problem for me and one week I was late clocking in for four days on the trot. The bosses would go really mad when you were late so on the fifth day I was determined to beat the system and clock in on time even though I was late again. After rushing off the bus, rather than go all the way around the factory to the main entrance, I jumped over the wall straight into the workshop. Unfortunately I had not taken into account the security system which, of course, triggered the alarm. As a result I was hauled in front of one of the directors for a right rollicking. Although I was looking to begin my career and wanted them to start me on a mechanical engineering apprenticeship, the firm would only offer me a job in the spot-welding department. Apprenticeships were as rare as hen's teeth and only two people out of the whole course were given those posts. So I ended up doing a job that was physically hard and very repetitive. It is the sort of boring work that is probably done by robots now and after about a year I came home and told my mum, 'I can't do this until I'm 65. It will kill me.' This decision was probably the best one I could have made at that point in my life. I did not want to be stuck in a factory; I wanted to live my dream.

Although I was on good money there, I told Stoves that I wanted to have another go at college so gave my notice in and started a BTEC Mechanical Engineering course at St Helens College. The management didn't want me to leave but I couldn't carry on. I realised that going to college was the only way I could fit in training and with less stress I could perform better on the field. I really didn't know what path I wanted to take, but I knew that one was not for me. Looking back, everything happens for a reason and maybe riveting all day probably did me a favour because I felt so lucky when I played rugby for a living. Knowing and experiencing what other people do in their daily lives for work – the people who paid my wages when I was playing – made me count my blessings when I was out on the park with a ball in my hand.

2

It's In the Blood

Having a professional rugby player as a dad undoubtedly influenced me in my interest in sport from a young boy and his guidance fuelled my quest to always give my best and be honest. My dad, Eric, had a long and distinguished professional rugby league career after signing for Saints from Widnes ICI rugby union club in 1968. Although he is best known for being a fiery back rower, he started off his career on the wing, and scored two tries in the three-quarters in Saints' 1970 Championship Final win over Leeds.

His performances caught the eye of the representative selectors, making the first of his 11 appearances for Lancashire in 1971. Unfortunately a shoulder injury meant he missed out on selection for Saints' 1972 Wembley winning side and not long after began looking for a move. My dad joined Salford at the start of the 1972-73 season for a world record £13,500 fee. That was big money back then – a record signing – and he enjoyed some great years there with that team they dubbed the Quality Street gang. There were household names galore at the then palatial Willows ground – including Keith Fielding of BBC's *Superstars* fame, former rugby union internationals David Watkins, Mike Coulman and Maurice Richards and seasoned international test players Steve Nash, Chris Hesketh, Ken Gill and Colin Dixon. He was successful, too, playing loose forward in Salford's glory years in the mid-seventies when they were Champions in 1973-74 and 1975-76, also winning the Lancashire Cup and BBC2 Floodlit Trophy in that time.

Although I was only little, I recall watching him play at Salford and also remember the antics me and Neil got up to. We used to sneak into The Willows club and play the drums and also run wild, recreating tries that we had witnessed from our heroes, unbeknown to my mum who was in the tea room. After winning the title in 1976, dad brought the magnificent old Championship trophy home and my mum still has photographs somewhere of me standing inside the cup in our back garden.

My dad must have left a lasting impression at Salford because as part of the celebrations to mark the closure of the Willows in 2011, a panel chose him as the best Red Devils loose forward to grace the old ground's turf. Of course in those days rugby league was a part-time profession, with training nights taking place after he'd done a full day's work as a painter and decorator for Widnes Corporation. Nevertheless he always gave it 100 per cent on the field, no matter what.

Salford's fortunes hit the slide in the late seventies but my dad's career was given a new lease of life when he got a transfer to Cup Kings Widnes in 1980 for £22,000. It was a great move for him and although he was very much in his veteran stages what a swansong he had there, partnering another veteran in big Cumbrian Les Gorley in the second row. There were big games galore with back-to-back Wembleys. A rejuvenated Chemics side beat Hull KR in 1981 with teenage scrum half Andy Gregory making a try scoring debut beneath the Twin Towers.

My dad brought the Challenge Cup home and I took it to show off at my St John Vianney junior school. In fact school had two Wembley winning dads that year with Widnes centre Eddie Cunningham's sons also at St John Vianney and we were all so proud of what our dads had done in front of a massive television audience. Wembley was the only time of the year when rugby league hit the back pages of the paper – it was massive. Bringing the cup home has its downsides as well as positive ones and my dad slept with trophy at the side of the bed because he was worried something would happen to it. I now know what he meant because when we won it in 1996 I brought it home and I locked that very same trophy up in our en suite whilst we slept.

We saw my dad play in some exciting games and I was getting old enough to understand what was going on but in 1982 there was a cup semi-final against Leeds at Swinton's old Station Road ground that proved a little too much – for my mum anyway.

Widnes were trailing the Loiners by three points with just a few minutes left on the clock and so it looked like Wembley was off that season. As the tension mounted, my mum began getting a little too worked up watching it and said; 'That's it!' and we had to leave because she couldn't watch any more. As we were walking out of the ground the crowd nearly lifted the roof off, but we did not know who was cheering. It turned out Widnes centre Keiron O'Loughlin had scored off a trademark Mick Adams up-and-under that took a bounce off the crossbar to make it through to Wembley again. So for two years running me, my nana and family friends went to watch my dad play beneath the famous old Twin Towers. They were good times to remember – and as an eight-year-old I supported the black and whites of Widnes.

Rugby was part of my weekly routine when I was growing up and I was a ball boy at Widnes' Naughton Park ground and then at minnows Runcorn Highfield when my dad crossed the Mersey for a final last hurrah with the oval ball. My brother Neil and I were even allowed to train at Canal Street when my dad was playing at Runcorn.

As a player my dad was quite physical – although he was not the biggest of blokes he threw himself about with scant regard for the impact on his body. I suppose he was quite a dirty player and used to get sent off. One day we all went to watch him play at Runcorn but arrived four minutes after kick off. We looked but my dad was not on the field – but a quick count up of the 12 players on the park indicated that he had already been allowed first use of the soap!

Another time he was playing for Widnes against Warrington – a big Cheshire derby and always something of a grudge match, especially in those days. When one of his opponents lost a boot in the tackle, my dad's first reaction was to pick it up and launch it out of the ground. That was the competitive streak in him – he was always quite involved, committed and deadly serious about his rugby.

Widnes played the all-conquering Australians in 1982 and my dad was giving it the works, walloping everything in green and gold. This 'Roos team was dubbed 'The Invincibles' but that night they must have thought it meant 'Untouchables'. Word had it that a message went out that if Widnes didn't take my dad off, because of the way he was carrying on, that they would walk off. My dad had a fight at half time during which one of the Aussies spat in his face. He went to reply in kind, but forgot he still had his gum shield in, so it just dribbled down his chin instead.

Rugby league back then was a different era. It was rough, tough and not as well policed as it is today – there was no video review panel, man in the stand or what have you. It was a physical environment and seeing him come home with cuts and bruises became the norm, part and parcel of his job, and he had lost all of his front teeth through rugby. Of course none of that remotely discouraged me from playing.

My dad is someone who I have always looked up to and he has been a great role model for me. My classmates at school were always asking me for his autograph, especially when he had been in a big game on television. Although that made me proud I never felt any different or better than the other kids in the class.

Playing tough, physical combat sport in the pack has left its mark on my dad. There were no conditioning and rehab sessions then after a game – just an early start back up the ladder painting and decorating. He is paying for it now and has a bad shoulder, back and neck. He played rugby for a long time – too long. Although he enjoyed the rough, tough stuff at the time and has run marathons since retiring they have subsequently discovered that he must have broken his neck playing – but he doesn't know when.

Understandably, I always followed Salford and Widnes as a boy purely because my dad was playing for them – just like my eldest son Taylor now supports Hull FC and Saints because they were my teams as a player. So my background, family and upbringing meant that rugby league was very much in my blood.

3

I Won't Back Down

People always told me that I was too small for such a high-impact, big collision sport as rugby but it never stopped me from playing and succeeding. In fact the doubters just made me more determined to prove them wrong. The opportunities just came along and it eventually resulted in me going down to the famous Knowsley Road of my hometown team with my dad to sign professional forms with Saints in 1992.

It was not an easy or straightforward path to get to that point. It all really began a few years previously when Danny Rylance started a junior rugby league team at Nutgrove. A couple of Saints directors, who watched me score three tries against Kippax, invited me to training up with the big guns of the first team at the front pitch at Knowsley Road. I was built like a stick and in a sport fixated on size I did not get signed up from that session, but fortunately there were other chances. One day, when I was having a kick-about in a side street near my home, former Saints captain Eric Chisnall pulled up in his car. Eric had played alongside my dad with Saints in the early seventies and he wanted to know if I fancied playing for the under 18s academy side he was setting up.

Of course, I jumped at the chance and ended up having a few games for the Saints under 18s. One game in particular sticks out – it was against the strong Wigan Academy at Knowsley Road. I can remember a young Jason Robinson playing in the stand-off position, he was outstanding, scoring four tries. It was evident at that young age that he was going to be a superstar. I played on the wing as my physical stature was more of a football player than a rugby player. My opposite number, Mike Neal, was much more developed than me; in fact at the time I thought he was enormous. He tried to knock me off my game with some old school sledging by shouting across, 'Prescott, I'm going to kill you!' It frightened me to be honest. Sure enough, when I got the ball on the wing he manhandled me into touch and I fell awkwardly, breaking my collar bone. I was straight off to hospital, still in my kit, and I still have the jersey from that day hung up in the loft. This was the first of many occasions when I doubted myself and wondered whether I was cut out for rugby league. It seemed I would never achieve my dream and follow in my father's footsteps.

At that stage in my career I was looking for a position – because of my natural pace they played me on the wing or at stand-off. After a year playing at the academy Frank Barrow, who was in charge of the Saints 'A' team, asked me to have a trial. But after playing a few games in the reserves as an AN Other, Saints told me they did not want to sign me, which was bitterly disappointing. Once again they believed me to be too small to make it.

It was a similar story at Widnes where, after one trial match at the old Naughton Park against Oldham, I was told by the coaches at the time I was no better than what they had already got in the 'A' team, the reserves. After facing rejection you have just got to get your head up, get on with things, knuckle down and try to make it somewhere else. Looking back I believe all these incidents made me a mentally stronger person and moulded the person I am today.

However, I have to thank coach Frank Barrow for persuading the board at Saints to give me another go. Frank had been a good full back in his day, winning every medal going in the all-conquering Saints side of the sixties, and must have seen some potential in me. He gave me the number one jersey for a few games.

Still the Saints board needed some convincing about what I was capable of, and it took Frank's genuine offer to pay my contract out of his own money to swing it. He really fought for me over this when others had doubts, and I will always be really grateful to him for that.

That summer I went to the gym and got bigger and stronger and Saints said, 'Ok – we'll give you a go in the 'A' team.' I actually signed for the club in November 1992. It was not a hugely lucrative contract, but it helped me greatly at the time because I was only a college student having packed in my job welding ovens. I was on £70 a win and £20 for a loss, which was a lot for me. Signing on the dotted line for Saints was one of the proudest moments of my life, especially since I was following in my dad's footsteps. My dad came with me for the signing and you could tell he was proud as punch. Although I was a realist and knew there was still a lot of hard work to do to progress through the ranks, I was nonetheless over the moon to be on the first step of the ladder.

I slotted in comfortably. All the 'A' team lads liked a drink and we used to knock about together and enjoyed the craic. However, it was when I was invited out with the old heads in the first team that the drink got the better of me. Saints' first teamers used to go out on what they called 'Tuesday Club' where they would go boozing around St Helens. Although I was still only a kid, I made the mistake of trying to match them pint-for-pint one night and ended up getting really drunk. Skipper Shane Cooper realised the state I was getting in and nudged me, saying, 'Listen son, it's time you got home,' but stupidly I shrugged him off. We ended up in Nabi's restaurant in Westfield Street by which stage I was already paralytic. There was no respite from the drink and as soon as we sat down Great Britain centre Paul Loughlin shouted, 'Pints of cider all round –down them in one!' We ordered some food, downed our ciders in one and then I stood up, staggered outside and fell over. After floating in a homeward direction, being shunned by every sensible taxi driver, I fell down hugging a lamppost and went through some bushes in the grounds of Pilkington Glass head offices. I must have just settled there because I woke up the next morning sniffing grass. It had been my first big night out with the Saints first team lads, but I spent the next day lying on the floor of my mum's bathroom being sick. It was a lesson learned.

Playing in the 'A' team was a good experience and I did well scoring lots of points which gave me a chance in the first team. Saints coach Mike McClennan was so impressed with me that he told the newspapers that I would be a Great Britain full back within three years.

There were some really memorable matches playing for that 'A' team, but the 13 against 13 fight at Batley sticks out. And sure enough our coach Frank Barrow was on the touchline cheering us on because he was a no-frills up and at 'em sort of coach who loved seeing his lads getting stuck in. That first year playing against men, not boys, was really tough and rugby league was all about size. It was difficult at first, but I could survive the bigger hits by using my powers of evasion and my natural speed. The more games I played, the better it became, with the experience helping me to know where to run. But there were a few moments along the way that made it something of a steep, and occasionally painful, learning curve. Against Halifax I went up for a bomb along with the massive former Welsh rugby union forward Paul Moriarty, who ended up smashing me head first into the floor – I didn't know what day it was. In another game I was hit so hard that I got up and played the ball facing the wrong way. The most bizarre injury I experienced was taking a bang to the head in the 'A' team game against Widnes. In the shower after the game, I did not even recall playing.

My confidence continued to grow and I was soon up there with the top point scorers from previous years. I was making the headlines in the local press and rugby league papers most weeks with my strong performances. This led to my first team debut against Leigh on September 19, 1993 even though I only played for the last three minutes. The next time was two months later, again starting on the bench at Headingley, but coach McClennan ended up pitching me in on the wing. Leeds were a big, physical side and I was still just a skinny lad, but I had my own individuality. My dad had given me some shoulder pads and as I strapped them on in the dressing room, wingman Anthony Sullivan said, 'You wouldn't need those pads if you did weights.' It felt like he was having a go at my size and it knocked my confidence a little.

A few days later I finally got to start against Oldham and all my mates from Thatto Heath came down to watch the game at the Watersheddings. My first points in senior rugby came that afternoon but bizarrely I also managed to kick the ball into my mate's face with a miscued conversion. My first try, quite fittingly in retrospect, came in the defeat against Hull at the Boulevard at the beginning of December.

The Saints team was on a bit of a losing streak under Mike McClennan but that probably gave me a chance of fulfilling my dream of playing first team rugby a little bit more regularly. Although assistant coach Frank Barrow tried to help my positional play, I was largely left to my own devices as a free running full back and it was a case of learning my own trade. Dave Lyon was Saints' number one at the time and one day, when he was out injured, I walked up to him and said, 'I'm not going away, you know.' I always regret saying that because it created a bit of tension between us and he must have naturally thought of me as an arrogant prick. Understandably he never really helped me, which I know now to be my own doing. I could have learned lots off Dave because he was a good full back, and model pro, but he probably thought I was too cocky. You have moments of weaknesses and that was one of them. Since my illness Dave has supported me and hopefully has forgotten and forgiven my teenage error.

That Saints team I had come into was playing poorly and as such the coach's days were clearly numbered. McClennan was shown the door when he threw a pint over a spectator during one particularly bad home defeat against Warrington. Eric Hughes, who had been the club's conditioner, took over the coaching reins. He had enjoyed a long distinguished career, and had played alongside my dad at Widnes. Eric brought in former rugby league referee Stan Wall as a conditioner. Some of Stan's training sessions had the lads in stitches – he had us doing bouncing stretches, which were unorthodox to say the least. Eric's big emphasis, however, was on youth coming through, so that was good news for me.

Apart from having pace as an attribute, my ability to strike a ball was an added string to my bow. Former Saints scrum half Neil Holding, who was the Knowsley Road groundsman at the time, agreed to open up and put the floodlights on to let me practise my goalkicking from the touchline.

Some things took some getting used to. For a start, when I broke into the first team, someone asked me for my autograph meaning I had to practise my signature. They were really good times and I was asked to open the new McDonald's restaurant on the St Helens Linkway. My name was in the *St Helens Star* every week – which sounds a small thing now, but it was all new to me then.

There were downsides, too, and it was not all plaudits and pats on the back and I soon learned that when you are put up there on a pedestal someone always wants to knock you off it. Playing out there with the first team I could hear fans shouting at me and in one game there was one bloke in the paddock section who was particularly abusive. He was shouting, 'Prescott, you wanker, couldn't tackle a Sunday dinner.' At the end of the game, I stood looking at him as he shouted, 'Come on!' whilst beckoning me towards him. It was hard to believe that this was a so-called Saints fan. Admittedly it wasn't one of my better games, but I was so close to going over into the paddock and getting hold of him. I can fully understand why, a few years later, Eric Cantona went into the crowd that time at Crystal Palace to karate kick the fan who was insulting him.

As a part of the team I was sociable with the players both from Saints and other teams. On some occasions I was perhaps a little too sociable and one night I went out to the Mr Smiths nightclub in Warrington with Paul Barrow and Iestyn Harris, who were both playing at the Wires at the time. After knocking back every cocktail on the list we began messing about outside and I decided to demonstrate that I was not as bad at tackling as some folk wanted to make out. After flattening them both with flying tackles, Paul got up and whacked me and I went straight through the back of a car window. Of course, it was not any ordinary window – it happened to be a police car! After I picked myself up and brushed off the glass I saw the eight police officers around me and I just said, 'Go on then, where's my seat?'

Paul bounded over to the car and said, 'It was my fault, let me in!'

It was quite funny when Paul was interviewed on tape down at the station – and was asked if there was any malice. He said, 'No, we were just prancing about like tigers!'

At the end of 1993-94, there was a crunch from my groin as I kicked for goal. It did not improve so I was sent to see Mike Scott, a specialist at Fairfield Hospital. He was using a revolutionary new technique to repair hernia damage using keyhole surgery and a type of mesh. The operation took place at the end of the summer and although the hernia had been repaired, they also found some multiple small bowel adhesions. This is basically where the bowel is attached to the stomach wall and the adhesions were a legacy of my earlier appendix surgery. Mike had tried to free these but was unable to because I must have been in some distress on the operating table. This hindered my recovery process and delayed my return to the field. The question has since been asked if this was a sign that all wasn't well within my abdomen.

Fortunately, though, I was still able to resume full training after three weeks and played in the fourth week. My aim was to continue progressing in the first team in 1994-95 and hopes were high that with new recruits Apollo Perelini, Scott Gibbs and Bobbie Goulding on board Saints were capable of challenging for honours.

Looking back I felt that the coaching staff had still not really made their minds up about me in the number one jersey. They had given me a few games the season before and I missed out at the end of the campaign. I was not picked to start the first game of the season, which Saints surprisingly lost at home to newly promoted Doncaster. The Dons had always been the sport's whipping boys and a decade earlier they had made a documentary about them – *Another Bloody Sunday* – on account of their miserable losing run. So to see them turn up at Knowsley Road and destroy a Saints side featuring three new star signings was a massive turn up. That shock result probably helped me, because I was back in the team the following week at full back. Although we lost that game 31-10 at Warrington, I was reasonably pleased with my own performance, but it was also significant for the lad who was making his debut that day – Keiron Cunningham.

Although I had started to make the breakthrough into the first team during the previous season, progression was never easy. However, the youngsters could now see that there was a pathway into the first team, but much of this was down to Eric Hughes. When he took over, youth came to the fore, giving them the opportunity to break into the first team. Eric was very much a hands-on type of coach – literally – he used to do the rub-downs in the dressing room before the match where he would give players instructions and motivation as he worked. However, he would certainly let you know when you failed to meet his expectations. He really lost his temper with us during one training session, where I guess the lads were not giving the session their undivided attention, and let us have it with both barrels, barking, 'You are a set of wankers. All you lot are interested in is shagging, Ford Probes and fucking mobile phones!'

The 1994-95 season was my second season in the first team at Saints, traditionally the hardest year for a player breaking in. Despite the possible difficulties of the 'second year syndrome', when opposition players and coaches have worked you out a bit more, it was good for me and I scored 20 tries. I was more off-the-cuff than the traditional full back and my game revolved around broken-field running. Everything was instinctive and I was lucky in that they gave me the licence to do it. Throughout my career I was never regimented too much by the coaches I played for and that was a major boost for me.

The stand-out game for me that year was against the touring Australians at Knowsley Road. Although it was the Kangaroos' midweek side they still had a cracking team and I was thrilled to have been awarded the man of the match award. The highlight was taking a few 'bombs' under pressure which meant the Knowsley Road faithful started to appreciate my efforts all the more. From that display I was selected for the Great Britain under 21s against Australia at Gateshead. We lost 54-10, with me scoring all the points, including a try from a grubber kick. When asked by a journalist who had most impressed him over here during the tour, the Kangaroos coach, Bob Fulton, came up with two names – Jonathan Davies and Steve Prescott. Fulton had seen me in the club game and the under 21s. Needless to say it gave me a real boost and later that season I was picked to play for the GB under 21s in the defeat against France at Albi.

There was further international recognition for me in early February, when I was named in the squad for the Coca Cola World Sevens in Australia. Even though it was a memorable experience to score at the Sydney Football Stadium against St George it was disappointing to go 12,000 miles to play just 28 minutes of rugby. It was crazy really.

Domestically our all too familiar foe Wigan were again the major obstacle stopping Saints from winning any major honours that year. We played them five times that season, drawing one and losing four. They ended our Regal Trophy hopes early in the New Year and it was inevitable that we would draw them again in the Challenge Cup fourth round. It wasn't a good day, with the torrential rain making it a wet and a muddy Central Park pitch, but we showed our potential by snatching a draw in front of BBC's *Grandstand* cameras. We could have gone out during the last few minutes when Wigan's Gary Connolly broke down the Douglas Stand side and almost aqua-planed towards the try line. However,

I threw my head, shoulders, chest and kitchen sink at him, flying into the hoardings, but the weight of my body managed to take his legs over the touchline. Dave Lyon picked me up off the floor and said, 'Brilliant, Precky…well done!' I didn't really know what had happened, but the touch judge had put his flag up. Alas the bubble of expectancy was burst by a big Wigan pin and we lost the replay 40-24 at Knowsley Road. A season that had promised so much ended with a Premiership semi-final defeat by Leeds.

Wigan looked as formidable as ever, but over the next 12 months their overall dominance – and the nature of the game of rugby league itself – was to change dramatically for everyone. In April 1995 the talk was of a 'war' basically between the Australian Rugby League and Rupert Murdoch's Super League for the right to televise rugby league. It also meant that the top British players would be offered huge loyalty bonuses to stay in this country instead of being targeted by the ARL. Towards the end of April Bobbie Goulding, Alan Hunte, Scott Gibbs, Sonny Nickle, Chris Joynt and I were called to meet the board at Knowsley Road where we were offered improved Super League contracts.

It was all cloak and dagger stuff. Joynty came down after his appointment and said he couldn't talk but asked if I knew anyone in the ARL who was interested in signing me. The only thing I could think of was what Bob Fulton had said in the press during the Australian tour. Anyhow, I went in and club directors Mal Kay and Tom Ellard told me that the club wanted to go full-time in the new proposed summer Super League. At the time I was earning around £15,000 a year, but Saints were offering a £25,000 contract, plus £10,000 in my hand for signing. They said that I needed to sign immediately because the offer wouldn't be available the following day.

It left me in a real dilemma and after leaving the meeting I tried to ring my agent, David McKnight, but his mobile was switched off. I didn't know whether to accept their offer or not so I asked my dad what I should do for the best. He told me to accept their offer, so I went back up and signed to become a full-time St Helens Super League player. Anyhow, I went away and finally managed to contact my agent, who apologised and said that he had been dealing with a lot of the Wigan 'A' teamers. McKnight said, 'You've not signed have you?' I told him that I had. He then told me that he had just got £50,000 cash for Wigan 'A' team lads, plus £50,000 contracts.

McKnight tried to get me out of the contract by saying I had signed on my own and had been pressured into it, but Saints were having none of it. On this issue I just felt that the directors didn't look after me. They could have helped me out and got me a bigger contract particularly as I don't think they were actually paying it – that was Super League. If I had got sorted then with a much-improved contract I would have probably stayed with Saints long term. That said, I can't grumble too much because I got £10,000, which helped me put a deposit down on a house.

Years later, when I was with Hull FC, I asked Jason Smith if he ever did the lottery. He turned to me with a smile before telling me what he received as a consequence of the ARL-Super League war was like winning the jackpot – and he has a fantastic penthouse next to the beach at Cronulla to prove it. Good luck to him. He was in the right place at the right time.

Just before our last league match of the season, I developed a really bad cough and took two spoonfuls of Benylin and some Buttercup Syrup so that I could get a good night's sleep. Perhaps I didn't fully realise the consequences at the time, but I played well the next day and was man of the match. After the match, I was drug-tested for the first time and suddenly thought 'Oh my God ... I've taken cough medicine!' Benylin contains pseudo-ephydrine, a stimulant, which is a banned substance in rugby league.

My sample went off for testing and a few weeks later they sent me a letter to appear at a disciplinary hearing in Leeds. I placed the bottle of Benylin on the desk and explained what I had taken. They passed the bottle around the table and they all looked at the ingredients. I told them I had been naïve, but that was all I had taken. They were prepared to let the matter rest with a stern warning, but the incident would go on my record for future conduct. There is no way that it could have improved my performance, of course, but the whole thing was a real wake-up call. Coincidently, the next two games saw me provide a urine sample in the 'random' drug test.

4

Following My Dream

Before we embarked upon the new Super League at the end of March in 1996, there was a special abridged Centenary season, with the World Cup tucked into it. The World Cup took place in October and, given the praise I had received from Aussie coach Bobby Fulton and my progress as an international player, I was really disappointed not to have been selected for the England World Cup squad.

Kris Radlinski was first choice for the full back jersey and he was really an exceptional player. We were obvious rivals on the field for our respective clubs, Saints and Wigan, but how could you possibly be bitter over a player like Radlinski? He remains one of the best blokes you could ever meet, whether you are rivals or not.

This game throws up different sorts of rivals – and by contrast, there was Lee Penny, Warrington's full back, who seemed to have a real downer on me. Although Kris and I were great rivals, we still respected each other and spoke to each other. Lee, on the other hand, adopted a completely negative attitude towards me – he played as if he hated me with a passion. He would come in with his knees when he tackled me and generally try to take my head off when I took the ball in. According to my close friend Paul Barrow, who played for Warrington at the time, his Wire team-mates had wound Lee up with tales about how I was coming to Wilderspool to take over his number one jersey, so that probably explains it.

Radlinski went on to play every match in the World Cup, with great success. Perhaps the squad was selected with Gary

Connolly and Jason Robinson as cover for the full back position – two more really world-class players there. It was still a massive disappointment to miss out on what was a great international event with a Wembley showpiece. I spent time analysing my game a bit more afterwards and once again I gathered that my two main weaknesses were in my defence and my physical size.

There were to be more changes on the horizon before that season was over. Shaun McRae, who was a renowned conditioner with Canberra Raiders and backroom member of the Australian World Cup squad, was invited by Saints' board to take coaching for a fortnight and I can say without hesitation that those two weeks were probably the most exhaustive I have ever experienced. Shaun must have thought, 'They're going to get everything I can throw at them!' He was there to impress and a hidden agenda obviously existed that we didn't know about at the time.

A rather disjointed season ended with us beating Warrington 80-0 before narrowly losing to Wigan in the Regal Trophy Final at Huddersfield's McAlpine Stadium. Wigan seemed invincible before that clash but our team of young lads certainly made it a contest. We were obviously really disappointed with the defeat, but looking back now, it was valuable experience for us and the perfect springboard for future success in Super League.

It was a pity that Eric Hughes did not last too long as coach because his youth policy had undoubtedly laid excellent foundations for the future of the club. He was very much a traditional type of coach and a great motivator, but not necessarily a technical coach, which is probably why Shaun McRae was brought in.

We were full time players in 1996 and rugby league was changing. Shaun was the first coach to introduce analysis of the opposition and our own game. We had never really seen this type of technical approach before. With Shaun we used to set ourselves goals and targets before the game and write down information on the opposition, together with an assessment of our own performance, rating ourselves out of 10 afterwards. He used to take the sheets away, mark them and give players his score. We heard he had previously been a school teacher, which made sense.

Shaun, who was nicknamed Bomber, put a whole emphasis on new conditioning drills that he had brought from Australia. He also introduced weight-training and we used to get occasional advice from Jack Penman, a weight-lifting champion. Jack emphasised the need for mental, as well as physical, strength, which had a profound effect on the team overall. Everybody enjoyed doing the weights, except our naturally gifted centre Paul Newlove, who hated the sessions. When we were in the gym we had an attitude that we never quit and kept going and that's what helped us in 1996. It gave us a focus as a team and as individuals to beat everything that faced us.

The Centenary season overlapped into the start of the Super League campaign and we did not get an off-season as such with our progress in the Challenge Cup which took us all the way to Wembley. In Bomber's first game in charge we hammered Castleford in the Challenge Cup at Wheldon Road and I scored a good try that helped kill them off. I caught a bomb near my own line, beat Tawera Nikau and set off and rounded Jason Flowers. It was good for me, with it being Shaun's first game, because it showed the new boss what I was capable of.

Challenge Cup Final week was a totally different experience for me, including the fitting of our suits. Bobbie Goulding, as captain, picked everything, including a rather retro-looking waistcoat that we all had grave doubts about. Still, it could have been worse. When we got to Wembley, we saw the Bradford lads out on the pitch and they were dressed in burgundy, like Wallace Arnold coach drivers.

As we lined up in the tunnel, in squad number order, I was second, behind captain Bobbie and Robbie Paul was right next to me. I was trying to focus and I was really fired up – after all, it was my first Wembley. Cool as a cucumber, Robbie kept spinning a ball on his fingertip but I was so psyched up I felt like knocking it out of his hands. They held us in the tunnel for a good few minutes and then the whole stadium erupted when we walked out. It sent a tingle all down my body and I sort of froze. We walked out to the middle to M People's 'Search for the Hero' and I felt so drained, my energy had gone and it felt like there was nothing in my legs. We shook hands and lined up for the National Anthem and set off for our positions. When we kicked off to Bradford I was still a nervous wreck. Somewhat surprisingly, Paul Loughlin immediately returned the ball with a down-town kick of his own. The ball dipped and bounced, and bounced again, and for that split second I was thinking, 'What if I knock on?' I managed to grab it and ran towards their defensive line. All my nerves seemed to disappear at that moment.

We made a good start and I was delighted to score our first try after just four minutes. It was a cross-field bomb, palmed back to me by Scott Gibbs giving me virtually a clear run to the line with 10 yards to go and I dived and slammed the ball down on the turf. I shot up immediately and flung my arms into the air. It was pure elation, realising that I had scored the first try on my first appearance at Wembley – a wonderful start to my greatest day in rugby league.

People say to me, 'You could have scored a hat-trick that day, if only the ball hadn't hit the crossbar' which is true. Bobbie and I had an understanding, where he would kick the balls and I would chase them and make them look good, although he would never admit that. On this occasion, I chased hard and was in a good position, I could challenge for a high ball, so I shouted to Bobbie, 'Aim for the crossbar!' He put the kick in and I leapt full length to get underneath the ball. Just when I was certain I was going to catch it, the ball hit the crossbar and bounced back. Bobbie and I have had some banter over that incident. He says I should have known how good his aim was and not told him to aim for the crossbar, although I'm not sure he could do it again if he tried.

Fifteen minutes later, I scored again and this was very much an off-the-cuff effort which had more than a little nod to my soccer days at Parr and Hardshaw. We worked the ball down the middle and I put my hand up for Bobbie. He would know instinctively that if he put it close to where I was running I had a reasonable chance of getting it. I said, 'Chip over.' Just as it came down I weighed up whether to let it bounce or catch it on the full. I decided just to volley it with my right foot and it went past the full back and as it bounced along the turf it hit my shin and bounced nicely over the line and I just dived on it.

A great start for me and the team but a quarter of an hour into the second half we were 26-12 down and needed to get back into the game desperately. It was time for Bobbie to launch his towering bombs that would produce three tries in seven minutes. Keiron scored the first, after the Bulls' full back Nathan Graham let the ball bounce. Then another kick went up – virtually identical – and Simon Booth got the ball down and a third for Ian Pickavance. We were back in the lead again and there was no stopping us after that.

Although it had been a closely-fought game, there was never any talk of defeat at any time during the match. We were being challenged but when the going got tough, we had the physical and mental strength to handle the pressure. From doing our work in the gym, we had it in our minds never to give in. We didn't quit.

Karle Hammond said to me before the final, 'If we win this cup, make sure you get next to Bobbie and you'll be on all the photos for all time.' That is exactly what we did. You cannot re-create that feeling of climbing those famous steps to lift the cup. It is an unbelievable moment. As we went on the lap of honour people were throwing scarves in celebration. A lady threw a teddy bear with the number one on its back over to me and I still have it to this day. The best feeling was seeing my mum and dad with their friends in the crowd. I had emulated my dad by winning the Challenge Cup and it was a really emotional time. I could see my dad's face and he was so proud.

The following day's homecoming felt like the whole of St Helens was celebrating with us – it was a fantastic occasion, by far the best I have ever experienced.

Nobody was allowed to be big-headed in our team in those early days of Super League – if they were, there would always be people who would bring them back down to earth with a bump. When wingman Alan Hunte brought his new Saab convertible to training our big Samoan enforcer Vila Matautia threw a great big clod of earth all of 30 yards and it thudded onto the bonnet, covering it with dirt. Dean Busby, who had joined from Hull before the start of Super League, turned up for his first session in his Ford Cosworth. Andy Northey took Dean's keys out of the changing room and put a dead fish in the radiator. For the next few weeks when Dean turned on his heaters or cold blowers he had this rancid smell of rotting fish and couldn't really work out what the problem was.

Dean must be the unluckiest rugby league player of all time. Even before Super League had started he had problems. At the time he was tipping the scales at 15 stones and the aim was for everybody to get bigger and stronger with weight training. Dean's target was 16 stones, so when he came back from his off-season break in Jamaica he began the new strength-building regime with us. The whole squad saw their power, strength and weight increase

– apart from Dean. After two months he had actually lost half a stone. Apparently he had picked up a bug on holiday that had put him behind everybody else.

After starting to impress in the Centenary season, Dean played at Castleford in the Challenge Cup and went down with medial ligament problems in his knee and was out for another 10 weeks. He gradually got back into full training and was ready for his comeback in the 'A' team. He told the first team lads to come and watch, but after about 10 minutes he left the field with an 80 per cent tear in the cruciate ligament of his other leg – another six months out. He came back in 1997 and played about nine games and the week before we went to Australia in the World Club Championship we were playing Oldham at Boundary Park. Joynty put his hand up to indicate he needed a rest and Dean went on to replace him. Joynty went towards the bench and even before he had put on his subs jacket Dean had dislocated his ankle and broken his fibula and tibia and torn all his ligaments, putting him out for eight-and-a-half months. If he's not the world's unluckiest rugby league player I don't know who is. All the lads used to take the piss a little bit, but he was so unlucky. Yet Dean was good for the club ... he was a really funny guy always telling jokes and he kept our spirits high. It all added to the camaraderie of the year.

Another guy who added to the mix at Knowsley Road was Australian signing big Derek McVey. He was a real wind-up merchant and would rile the local lads with his talk that everything was much bigger and better back home. Even the stars were much brighter Down Under. Apart from his occasional moans, Derek was a powerful player, who could off-load the ball brilliantly and was a real star turn for us in the early days of Super League.

Our first home Super League game was against Wigan and was a must-win affair and early on there was a massive ding-dong at the scrum between Adam Fogerty and Neil Cowie. You really would not want to get between those two when they were going at it hammer and tongs, especially with Adam being a former boxer. Wigan led at half-time, although we knew we had the confidence to take them on and beat them. It finished 41-26 with Tommy Martyn coming off the bench and scoring a typically brilliant try to turn the game our way.

Apart from writing down the strengths and weaknesses of our

opponents in team meetings, coach Shaun McRae would make sure that everyone had an area of responsibility within the team framework. As full back, I had to do defensive adjustments during the match. He was giving players a responsibility ... it was like teaching. Other players had to shout out the tackles.

I was happy with my form but I was always someone you would describe as a confidence player. In the game against London Broncos I made a tackle and then moving to my right to make another, only for Greg Barwick to step out of it and score. Brian Case, who was running messages at the time, came out and said, 'Bomber says get your act together ...'

I was already fuming with myself mentally, so didn't need that and said: 'Brian, tell Bomber to fuck off!' Next thing the card was up from the touchline – number one, off you come. It kind of taught me a lesson. He substituted me for dissent and it was a kind of a wake-up call. I grew up as a result. Although I didn't mean for Brian literally to tell him, but he did – cheers Brian!

There was no let-up, with tough matches every week and another real test of our character as a team came when we faced Warrington at Wilderspool. It was probably one of the best games I have ever played in. The game was so tense, because we needed to keep winning with Wigan breathing down our necks. The sheer pressure of the situation motivated us that season and this particular game was a good illustration. I scored early on when I took the ball out of Lee Penny's hands from one of Bobbie's pin-point bombs.

It was a real ding-dong battle and we trailed 24-17 when Alan Hunte went through on an inside ball from Tommy Martyn and was stiff-armed by Penny, who was sent off. Five minutes from time Ian Pickavance played a 'one-two' with Derek McVey and stormed under the sticks for a brilliant try, which with Bobbie's conversion gave us the winning 25-24 lead.

The Castleford game was another crucial moment that maintained our league position. Towards the end of the match at Wheldon Road, we were leading 20-16 but under a bit of pressure when Jason Flowers looked like making the line. Both Joey Hayes and I tackled him virtually at the same time and he went down short of the line. It is considered one of the 'champagne moments' of the season and one that finally helped us to lift that first Super League title.

We thrashed Warrington, hitting the 60 mark again, on the last day of the season to win the Super League just ahead of Wigan. We had achieved a memorable cup and league 'double' – the first from a Saints' team for 40 years.

Somebody stamped on my hand and it swelled to a big lump so I came off before the end. I had to use my left hand to shake hands during the trophy presentations. Although the season was not over, it was celebration time. All the team were out that night and we took the trophy with us around St Helens, beginning at the Bird I'th Hand just up the road from the ground. The trophy was dropped somewhere along the way and the club had to get the dent fixed before returning it, but to go out drinking with it was something else. The 1996 season is the highlight of my career and it was a privilege to be in such a high-achieving team.

The early part of the summer of 1996 was dominated by football. Baddiel and Skinner's 'Three Lions' set the backdrop for Euro '96 which was held in England. Football may have been coming home but I had international landmarks of my own in June 1996. That is when I achieved another ambition by making my full England debut against France at Gateshead, kicking seven goals, scoring two tries to win the man-of-the-match award and establish an England individual points record of 22 in a match. It was a record that stood for many years.

My second game for England was a try scoring appearance against Wales at Cardiff Arms Park and those displays helped me secure Great Britain selection for the Oceania Tour at the end of the season. I was one of eight Saints' players picked for the tour, which was an indication of our dominance of that maiden Super League competition.

The Great Britain boss was Phil Larder, who I didn't rate really as a coach despite his big reputation, but he seemed to have a high opinion of himself. When being selected to tour you think you've got every chance of playing, but I sort of knew before I went that Steve Prescott would not feature in this coach's plans. You may ask why. Well, in the training session before we flew out, whilst standing on the sideline to interchange during an unopposed ball session, I heard the shouts 'Dave, Dave, Dave!' from Mr Larder. This was the Great Britain coach who was standing in the middle of the pitch, looking in my direction. Well I didn't get many qualifications at school, but even I knew that Dave wasn't my name and quickly looked over my shoulder to see if anybody was behind me. John Bentley, who was standing next to me, said 'I think he's talking to you.'

I replied quickly, 'But my name isn't Dave.' Can you imagine the fits of laughter between us and the look of confusion on Phil Larder's face? I was totally embarrassed and I still shake my head in disbelief now. I have since looked up Phil Larder MBE on the internet and found lots of quotes he has used during his coaching career. This was one: 'It's no surprise to me that fundamental skills are breaking down. One of the things put on the sidelines is work on basic skills. The breakdown of those skills has been a major factor in the losses.' However, to me fundamentals and basic skills would involve learning somebody's bloody name!

We flew to Papua New Guinea first and we were met by hundreds of people. It was a real eye-opener for us. The people there were addicted to this thing called beetle nut, which had rotted their teeth and had made their gums all red and swollen. We were told it had traces of cocaine in it, hence the addiction. It was really strange to see them smiling at us when we got off the plane. There didn't seem to be any made up roads on the way to our hotel, which was literally next to the rainforest. I played in the first game of the tour, against a PNG Presidents XIII at Mount Hagen and kicked five goals. They might have been small guys, but they certainly put themselves about in the tackle. I wasn't selected for the First Test at Lae, and even though it was obvious that I was going to be one of the 'ham and eggs', or the dregs, as we called ourselves on the tour, I enjoyed the experience of Papua and then it was on to Fiji. I was in the side that beat the Presidents XIII 42-16 and once again kicked five goals. There was also a Test Match at Nadi three days later, which Great Britain won 72-4 but was marked by the biggest brawl I have ever seen at any rugby match. It took referee Jim Stokes quite a while to restore order. Iestyn Harris threw a punch, got chased and was eventually decked. It was a brutal affair. Even big Brian McDermott – an accomplished boxer himself from his army days – was put down. A few moments after things had seemingly settled down, one of their players ran straight towards Bobbie Goulding with his fists up. I thought, 'Here we go, it's going to start again here.' As he ran towards him, Bobbie casually ducked to one side and belted him full in the face – but the Fijian kid was sent off for inciting more violence! It was surreal.

In New Zealand I played in Wellington against a Presidents XIII and the Maoris in Whangarei. Seeing the pre-match Haka, with their tongues out and their eyes almost popping out of their heads, was frightening in itself. I scored a try and kicked three goals in that match, although we were thumped 40-28.

Throughout the tour I had the impression that the Great Britain management were more interested in the Test match squad and I didn't enjoy the segregation of the two camps. We were away for six weeks, all told, but there was a sting in the tail. They ran out of money and so flew several of us home shortly after the match against the Maoris. We were dumped in London, after flying economy class all the way home, and they expected us to travel four hours on a coach back up north. In the end we paid for our own connecting flight back to Manchester.

Those of us on international duty did not get much in the way of off-season, but naturally we wanted to maintain our success in 1997 and made great strides in the defence of the Challenge Cup. We started off by beating Wigan at Knowsley Road – a good performance – considering we played for a large part of the game with 12 men after Bobbie Goulding had been sent off for a high tackle.

We again made it through to Wembley but the week before I scored when we beat Castleford at Anfield. David Howes knew of my interest in soccer and I was invited to help with the pre-match publicity, which included getting our photographs taken in front of the Kop with some of the Liverpool players.

I wasn't really nervous before the final but I had dropped a ball in that last game before Wembley which led to a try. That wasn't me. I was always confident in catching the high ball – renowned for it in fact. It was the sort of error I didn't need leading up to the final and it really dented my confidence, so I made sure I had a rugby ball with me virtually all the time at the hotel. I even slept with one to get my confidence up.

At Wembley our half backs Tommy Martyn and Bobbie Goulding dominated the match with their superb kicking skills. I went on an 80 metre break from a scrum virtually under our own posts. I did a sort of 'in and away' move on my opposite number Stuart Spruce.

This was a tactic I used in Super League with great success. Players seemed to plant their feet and my pace took me round them. The line wasn't getting any closer and although I had beaten Robbie Paul, Matt Calland and Abi Ekoku hit me simultaneously, tackling me into touch. I looked up, could see the line and couldn't believe I hadn't scored.

We had lifted the Challenge Cup for two years on the trot and I suppose the team – including me – had got a little too big for our boots. We thought we were invincible and needed knocking down a peg or two. Looking back some of the things we did after that game were totally unacceptable. In the post-match celebrations someone threw a tomato juice over a sponsor's wife after she told him to pick the top of the cup up off the floor.

Back at the hotel and the post-match reception we were all there, everyone in high spirits, getting drunk. Two fire extinguishers were let off during the night, which was just a case of young lads doing things without thinking. When we were on the coach back home, one group thought it would be funny to challenge some of the boys to pull a moony – basically drop their trousers and press their bum cheeks against the window to the next coach that came past us. They did it in good style, but to their shock, horror and amazement, it was a club coach that passed with all the directors and their wives on board. The catalogue of indiscretions continued when we got back to St Helens on the open-topped bus. We had been drinking all night and we were still drinking the following day. A woman came out of a house, shouting, 'Well done, lads!' Someone rather misguidedly gave her the finger and some verbal abuse. Then we found out that she was a Police Inspector's wife.

Before the next training session we were summoned by Eric Ashton and he had a long list of misdemeanours. It is an understatement to say he wasn't very happy:

- Item 1: Abuse of a sponsor's wife.
- Item 2: £500 cost of letting off fire extinguishers.
- Item 3: Making obscene gestures on the coach (mooning).
- Item 4: Abuse of a Police Inspector's wife.

Unfortunately, as the list of items was being read out by the chairman, there was the occasional smirk but by the final item, everybody burst out laughing. Of course, the incidents weren't funny, but it was just the way he had read them out. The chairman went absolutely ballistic and threatened us all with getting the boot from the club. Needless to say we paid for the damage. We were celebrating our success in a team environment, but clearly we had gone over the top and deserved what we got. I can honestly say that I was not the culprit of any of the above items ... but I do know who was.

Things went a bit pear-shaped after the Challenge Cup Final. There was a massive injury list and there were perhaps other factors that contributed to our slump. Maybe we liked the high life too much and lacked discipline on occasions. The World Club Championship came just in the middle of our injury crisis, which didn't help matters. The first three games were at Knowsley Road and we were well-beaten in all three against Auckland Warriors, Cronulla and Penrith.

It was then that my groin problems flared up again and the only option was to have a surgical procedure to repair and reinforce the previous injury. There was also a problem with the abductor muscles, which further complicated my recovery. Despite this, I still went on the plane for the return legs of the World Club Championship. Given our injury situation, there was a chance that I could possibly play in one or two of the matches down there. We decided to have a bit of bonding beforehand and quite a number of us bleached our hair blond. In retrospect it was one of the worst decisions we ever made – an absolute nightmare. We all had a pact that we would do it, but some relented when it was time to get it done. So there we were at Cronulla and the television cameras panned across the subs bench and everyone had bleached blond hair. Needless to say we were getting beaten and I wondered what the headlines would be like back home. We looked like real party boys, but we only did it to try to keep up our spirits as a team. The blond hair was simply an effort to bond us as a team, to try to be as one.

We stayed at the Holiday Inn at Coogee Bay and I roomed with Tommy Martyn, who was also not in contention for selection at this stage of the tour. It was quite tempting to go out and have a few drinks and so when we were given a night off and told we couldn't have a drink, we had a glass of lemonade in front of us, with a beer round the corner of a post. Every time we had a sip of the beer it was 'beat the system!' The first night we went out, I returned quite early. I was in the hotel room when the phone went. It was David Howes. I knew he was checking up on Tommy, who hadn't returned, so I had to pretend to be a Leyther. The ruse lasted all of three seconds before my cover was blown. 'That's you isn't it Precky? Where's Tommy?' I had to come clean and say I hadn't seen him, but it was worth a try.

On another night, we were allowed to go out, but had to be back by midnight. Some of us went out for a few beers, but we all reported back at different times. I suppose we thought that we were all high and mighty and wouldn't get caught, but all they did was to look at the electronic keys and we were in for the high jump.

We had to report to the Board the next morning. Apollo Perelini was the player's rep at the time and he came in with us. We were all fined £1,000 – a lot of money in those days. Chris Morley, in particular, was incensed at the outcome. He piped up, 'That's fucking disgraceful!' and stormed out of the room. Although we had broken the curfew, Tommy and I thought that we should not have got the same punishment, but they came down hard on all of us. Perhaps it was a throwback to our Wembley antics. We were young lads and if you are given the opportunity to get away with something, you will do it!

Having been given clearance to play in the second game in New Zealand I rang the specialist and explained that I was still sore. He said, 'Start training and see how you go.' I trained on the Wednesday ... after many months out and we were up and down on the field. I was shattered after a really tough session but later on Bomber said, 'You're playing.' I couldn't really believe it after so long out, especially against such a tough team as Auckland Warriors. I played and wished I hadn't. They put 70 points on us. I remember catching their stand-off, Gene Ngamu, with a cracking hand-off and away he went on his backside. I spent the bulk of my time on the field trying to chase people down. Lee Oudenryn, who was a real speedster, broke through. Bearing in mind I had returned from a groin op with virtually no training, no sprint work or anything like that, I ended up chasing him. I looked up at the screen, saw myself running and thought, 'What the hell am I doing on this field?' Shaun obviously knew what I was thinking and he brought me off shortly afterwards.

The day before the next match against Penrith we were doing some unopposed drills at Belmore Oval. Longy passed this ball to me and it was round my ankles. So I went down to catch it and I heard this crunch in my groin. My partial abductors had snapped away from the bone. Our physio Jeanette Smith wasn't exactly sure what it was at the time, but it turned out that I would never play for the Saints again.

People only tend to remember the hammerings that the British sides received during the World Championships, but it gave everyone a taste of what it is like to play at a higher level, especially those who didn't play internationally. It was also an eye-opener in terms of the facilities offered by Australian and New Zealand clubs for training players. We had only been full-time for 18 months or so when we went over there. It showed British clubs what we had to do to try to raise our standards. If they did it again now, things might be different. Rather than have every Super League club involved, perhaps they could have had a top six or top four competition at the end of the season, alternating between Britain and Australia.

Coach Shaun McRae gave me some time off for the close-season. I went on holiday to the Bahamas with Chris Morley, Sean Long and our partners. You can imagine what that was like, and although we had a great time, playing sport, relaxing on the beach and even scuba diving to the shipwreck from the James Bond film *Thunderball*, a decision to hire jet skis almost meant we nearly never came home.

One of the days we set off on jet skis and ignored all the warnings not to advance past certain points; we sped off into the distance. There were islands out there, which we took off for and then suddenly really big waves started coming up. We rode them at first for a laugh, but I remember looking over my shoulder and seeing Longy take off on a wave, more than 30ft in the air screaming, 'Yee haa!' like a cowboy. He bailed out, his jet ski was upside down in the water and he couldn't turn it over. I turned around once again and to my horror saw Chris also turned over and struggling too. I was then hit by a wave and flipped the same as the others. We were stranded, miles out to sea with big waves smashing into us. I dread to think what was lurking beneath us. We were in big trouble; the signs on the nearby island said, 'Beware!' Luckily, a break in the waves allowed me to get back on my jet ski and with a bit of help, Mozzer also managed to get his jet ski upright. We managed to tow Longy's jet ski to the island. By this time the guys from the beach came to look for us as we had been gone for so long. I still can't believe to this day that we managed to get back safely.

5

Across the Pennines

It is not usually a good sign when you pick up a newspaper and read that you are being linked with a move. But on my return from the Bahamas the papers had me lined up with a transfer to Hull. Saints had just bought Paul 'Patch' Atcheson and Paul Davidson on free transfers from Oldham Bears, who had gone belly up and had lost their place in Super League. Patch had been an international full back in his Wigan days, so it was a worrying time for me.

I wanted a higher contract. In rugby league you are lucky if you can play at the top level for 10 years. You have to get your life sorted as best you can for the good of your family. If you are not getting the money, you can't sort your life out – simple as that. Saints offered me £38,000 to stay at the club. The big earners, like Bobbie Goulding and Paul Newlove, were probably on six figures and there was no salary cap at the time. You didn't know exactly what other people were earning; I only knew that they didn't really pay local lads well at the time.

In 1996 I had played for England twice and toured with Great Britain; Saints had won the Challenge Cup and the Super League and I was still on £25,000. I just wanted a half-decent wage to reflect what I had done in the game and for them to show that they recognised what I had achieved as a local lad. That would have been more than enough for me. What they offered was quite a lot of money in those days, but compared to the others, it wasn't very much. I had some dissatisfaction because I didn't feel as though the club was looking after me. For me back then, £50k was a benchmark

– and if I was not going to get it from them at this stage, then I was never going to get it at Saints.

I was gutted by the whole situation because I had come up through ranks and Saints was everything to me at the time. I was born, raised and gone to school in St Helens. It was where I had learned my trade, I was St Helens through and through. It annoyed me at the end and I was really upset how it played out in the media. There was all this talk in the press that 'Prescott wants away' when in reality I just wanted a fair contract and was upset that they would not give it to me.

There was speculation about my situation in the press and one day, after a weights session, I saw Shaun McRae at the front of the club next to the training pitch and I asked him, 'Do you want rid of me at this club, what's going on?'

He said, 'It's not me,' and denied any knowledge of it. Obviously there was a bit of truth in it.

I first heard of Hull's interest while playing snooker in the bar at Saints when former player Steve Peters, who knew Hull coach Peter Walsh, asked, 'Do you fancy going to Hull?'

At one stage, the proposed move to Hull was virtually cut-and-dried. I was in talks with them, but a couple of days before the deal was going to go ahead, I got a phone call to meet Saints' Director Mal Kay the next day at 8.30am at the Little Chef on the East Lancashire Road. As I sat down, Mal Kay said, 'You don't have to go ... we don't want you to go.' Now I didn't know what was happening! Why was he telling me this when they had already arranged a deal? During the meeting, Mal took a phone call from my agent, David McKnight, who I had not had dealings with for a while. He was on the phone to Saints and had brokered a deal with Hull. They had sorted the deal out. He was talking to Mal about the deal being on while I was there!

Mal ended the call and said: 'You've caught me – you know what's happening now.' But I still had not a clue what was going on. I was only a kid, but I knew they were playing games and the deal was virtually done. So that gave me the impetus to tell chief executive David Howes that I was not going anywhere unless I got a better deal at Hull.

It is still a mystery to me to this day what they were playing at. I was upset to be honest and had a go at them. Nor could I figure out whether they were the good guys or bad guys. Thinking about it now still leaves a bitter taste in my mouth.

In the end I got what I wanted. I think Saints may have paid the extra money on my contract, to ensure the deal went through. Although I didn't want to leave Knowsley Road, I was off to Hull, together with Alan Hunte and Simon Booth and buoyed with the best contract of my career. The Saints' board had seen over £300,000 come in for the three of us and the money would be used to finance a deal for the young Warrington loose-forward Paul Sculthorpe. I have to say, I think Saints spent the money wisely.

Hull Sharks had just been promoted into Super League and Huntey was their big signing. Like me, Alan didn't really want to leave Saints unless the money was right for him. From my point of view, there was this nagging feeling at the back of my mind that I had just been thrown in as part of the deal to get Alan to join Hull. Steve Crooks, Hull's assistant coach told the club's management exactly what they would be getting when they signed me and said my arrival would be a great benefit for the team.

It was a new start for me – rugby is rugby no matter where you play it. It was tough for those first two years at Hull because I could see Saints were still winning things. It got to me a little bit because I could have still been there. But I moved on, made new friends and that is the fantastic thing about playing rugby league. It was tough leaving my family and friends behind in St Helens, but you have to go where your job is. It was only an hour and 45 minutes across the M62 in the car, so it was not the end of the world. There were some fantastic people at Humberside and, looking back, we made great friends there. From a social point of view Hull was the best club I have been at, even if it was a little strange uprooting my life to move there.

From signing it was straight into pre-season training, which was much tougher than at Saints – quite different and a lot more intense. Conditioner Mick McGurn, academy coach Steve Crooks and coach Peter Walsh were all involved in the sessions. The hardest thing for me was the rowing because I had never done that before. Mick, who later became the Irish rugby union conditioner, really made us work hard. In one session he made us all row for 5,000 metres and then do 12 laps of the oval and then back on the rowing machine for another eight 150s. It was new for me and really intense, so much so that Linzi told me that I disturbed her one night as I was rowing in my sleep. The players and staff at the club were very welcoming and happy to have us in the team – the club were in Super League for the first time and I think our signings had given them a lift. All the squad accepted us.

Prior to joining I had already learned that Hull fans are good to have on your side. When I was playing for Saints at the Boulevard I was going down the steps after the game and fans were spitting and throwing coins at us. We were on the losing side that day too – that was my first impression. I later learnt it is so much different being on the opposition than playing in black and white at the Boulevard. The fans were exceptionally passionate and gave me, personally, lots of support.

During the course of that season, we won eight games in the league, which is not bad. We finished above Warrington, and two points behind Wembley winners Sheffield. Ninth out of 12 was a good year as far as we were concerned.

For me, 1998 was a great season and I collected plenty of awards on the presentation night, including player of the year, the fans and vice presidents awards. The move had paid off for me and the fans liked me, probably because I returned the ball really well from kicks that year, scored some great tries and always gave my all. Tackling was not my best asset, but at full back you look good if you get it right. I was not the biggest bloke and missed a lot of tackles, but learned to do things to help me.

So we were happy with our performances – and so too must have been the coach. Peter's only downfall was that he was too sociable and too down to earth. The camaraderie at the club was great and Peter liked to drink with all the players. We had loads of nights out when we first went to Hull and got drunk regularly, but that made us closer together and team spirit was unbelievable. The most memorable of nights came after the Saints away game when we went to Widnes and basically got paralytic. It was absolute carnage, with a lot of people taking their clothes off and running around the pub naked. The funniest thing about it was at that time Peter Walsh was trying to recruit Karle Hammond, suspecting the loose-forward's nose may have been pushed out by Scully's arrival at Saints. The idea was to talk to him and his dad – but half an hour later the coach and conditioner was running round the pub semi-naked. Karle ended up signing for London Broncos!

Hull itself was a vibrant sporting city and we mixed a fair bit. We used to see Mark Hateley, who was then Hull City's manager, and some of the football lads. Respected boxing coach Steve Pollard took us for sessions in the gym. One day Pollard was preparing a boxer for a big fight, so he wanted to get his guy's face hardened by punches and enlisted our squad's help. It was quite brutal, but he got all forwards to take it in turns in the ring with this guy. Imagine Jason Timu, Hitro Okesene and all our big lads giving this bloke a pounding. His face had already taken a bit of pummelling, with red marks all over it, when Jim Leathem got in the ring and began teasing him. Jim was the joker in the pack and was doing the Ali shuffle and twirling his arms to taunt him. It was too much, this proud boxer had had enough and simply put a jab out and punched Leathem right on the nose. This bloke could take a pounding but he was not about to have the mickey taken out of him by us. It was funny – and all the lads were cheering.

After a good first year in Super League, Hull's recruitment of players for 1999 just didn't work out – replacing Hitro Okesene, Maea David, Jason Timu, Brad Hepi and previous year's star signing Alan Hunte put a major strain on the squad. Those who replaced them for what should have been a season of consolidation were not as effective, which undid all that good work and we went backwards. Some players carried injuries and others didn't even play at all. There were some good blokes in there, particularly Australian hooker Andy Purcell and Karl Harrison. Although Harrison was good player and leader, he was coming to the end of an illustrious career and was now a bit slower. It was his last year as a player and he went into coaching afterwards but I am glad I experienced playing with him.

Matt Calland made an immediate impression on the club captain Gary Lester during a pre-season booze-up in Hull. After walking into the bar toilet I found Matt holding Gary upside down above the toilet bowl, then continuously dunking his head in the water. Another newcomer was big New Zealand international forward Michael Smith, who had some odd traits. He used to carry a bum bag around everywhere with him and after training he would wait until everyone had got out of the shower before getting in. He was hot and cold in game and if he didn't fancy it he would not play. Early in the season, Smith played in the Challenge Cup tie at Castleford in a game we were all really up for. Smith, our big signing and impact player, was on the bench and he had only been on for a few minutes when we saw him on floor with his hand up saying, 'Get me off, I can't go on any more!' I thought he must have picked up a pretty bad injury. Driving home from Cas the story came out, and people added to it, that Smith had been out till the early hours drinking before a big game. He lost all credibility and the fans jokingly started singing, 'We're on the piss with Michael Smith!' at subsequent games that season. But Smith had let us down badly on this occasion – especially with it being a cup game.

Walsh was a good coach, but the team could not adapt to his concept of three ball players. He had the ideas, but had made some wrong signings to execute that and as a consequence results were poor. Walsh went and Academy coach Steve Crooks, who knew all about his lads coming through, took over. However, Crooks did not get off to the best of starts. In his first week he called a meeting under the Threepenny Stand for all the players and brought motivational speakers in. It began when Crooksy got his flip chart out, now I am not sure exactly, but there were four categories – player, bystander, terrorist and corpse. The player category was for players who had done everything that was expected of them. The bystander was for players who let others do things for them rather than them stepping up themselves. The terrorist was a category for players who had lots to give, but all in the wrong direction – they did not help the team. Finally, the corpse was for players who failed to offer anything. Steve put everyone from the team into a category. I was a 'trier' and had had a fairly good season, but I understood what he was getting at when he put me in the category of someone who could do a lot more, a bystander. He declared that I was happy to let things go by me and not change them. There were a few of us in that category.

Only one or two, including Andy Purcell, were put into the rank of 'Player'. If you were in one of those two categories you were considered to be okay.

Things took a turn for the worse when Graeme Hallas realised he was being placed in the Corpse category. He immediately stood up and as calm as you like just said, 'That's ok because I think you're a prick!'

Steve replied just as calmly, 'I think you had better go'.

Graeme stood up and responded, 'Don't worry, I'm going'. And he did. That was the last we ever saw of him at the club. It was a very bizarre situation and not a great start to the meeting. It was weird how calmly it all happened and how everybody found it so amusing when it was so serious.

But a row really erupted when he put Michael Smith in the bottom 'Corpse' category too. He tried to put up a defence, but all the lads were laughing at him. Then for some reason Crooksy put Steve Craven in the same category. Craven was a hard man; the sort of quiet bloke who just put his head down and kept going. He was outraged and jumped up shouting, 'How dare you put me in the same group as that knob head over there,' pointing his finger in the direction of Michael Smith.

Smith immediately jumped up and barked, 'Who are you calling a knob head?'

Andy Purcell then leapt out of his seat in Craven's defence and said, 'You had better sit down or I'll put you down!' This was our first training session under Crooksy and we walked away thinking, 'Oh dear, this is going to be fun.'

Later that year I dislocated my elbow at home to Huddersfield after I stretched out my arm to try to get the bouncing ball. They took me off on a stretcher and straight to hospital. I was in so much pain they put me to sleep to manipulate it back in. Believe it or not after all that, a fan had a go at me, saying, 'All you had to do was stretch out and you'd have scored.' I tried to explain that my arm was dangling at the time. They put me in plaster which meant once they took the cast off my arm was stuck at 90 degrees. In an effort to stretch the tendons and get movement back in the joint, physio, Keith Warner used to swing off my arm as part of my rehabilitation. The arm never fully recovered and even today it is two degrees out from being straight.

Perhaps my elbow was the least of my worries. Shortly before I returned to action we were hit with a bombshell, owner David Lloyd told us that the club was in financial difficulty and we weren't getting paid. Steve Crooks called us in for a meeting and he said we were all going to be on the equivalent of £25,000 a year for the rest of the season. Hull were in danger of being relegated and we were joint bottom with Huddersfield going into the last game of the season. It was down to a winner takes all because if we won our last game at home to Sheffield we would stay up. The headline in the *Hull Daily Mail* said Lloyd was going to give us all a grand a man if we won. We wanted to stay up anyway, even without the financial incentive, and when we hammered the Eagles, the Boulevard crowd was so happy they invaded pitch at the end because we had stayed up. Some Black and White diehards compared it to the championship winning exploits of 1983. Even though it was possibly the worst of seasons they carried the players off in celebration. It was unbelievable.

As it was, we never got that grand off Lloyd, so that 80 minutes of trying hard, though pleasing as a player, was not really rewarded financially. We got somebody to write Lloyd a solicitor's letter but he apparently said it was not his debt, and it had been passed on to the club. I had no time for Lloyd and the fans felt the same way. At one televised game there was a scrum and a protest group threw tennis balls on to the pitch. It was really funny, and they had to come on to clear them off. The upshot was the fans wanted him out of the club and he upped and left.

As for my career, there was talk that Gateshead, Castleford and London were supposedly interested in me. Hull were trying to find new money men and there was speculation that there was £1m on the table if Hull merged with Gateshead. It was all academic to me, because if you haven't got a deal you have got to go and get one sorted. My contract was null and void so I could not wait to see if the merger was going to happen. As it was I ended up getting some of the money I was owed when they finally merged and got their £1million. I was not bitter with Hull and I carried on living in the city when I signed for Wakefield Trinity Wildcats because we were settled there and loved the life we were living.

6

Trinity

When things went pear-shaped at Hull, I weighed up my options and after considering other offers, including one from Castleford, I opted for Wakefield Trinity Wildcats. Basically, I needed a club and was just glad of being able to get a bit of security for my family at that time. In financial terms, it didn't matter which club I was going to end up at, as I was going to be taking a huge pay cut no matter where I was going. This was the first time in my career that I realised how insecure a job rugby league can be. I remember people saying, 'Don't worry, you'll get another contract'. That maybe the case, but who will pay the mortgage in the meantime? You tend to live to your means and when that is taken away it can be a very worrying time.

Wakefield had been cut out of the original Super League line up when it was set up in 1996, but had won promotion in 1998 – and against the odds they stayed up in 1999. After that one season they decided that they wanted to kick on from there. They splashed the cash and the deal was sold on that there was some money in this club and they wanted established players. I guess that was me at that time. They were trying to move up the ladder by spending money – and with that they had big plans for developing their outdated old ground.

After years in the doldrums, Wakefield seemed to have found a pot of gold at the end of a rainbow and were throwing cash around bringing in, among others, Bobbie Goulding, England international Steve McNamara and promising youngster Ryan Hudson. Francis

Maloney and flying rugby union convert, Paul Sampson also joined the list of new recruits.

With Steve McNamara also living in Hull, the club figured I could travel over with him every day, even though at that time I did not know him. Steve and I had some really interesting journeys across the M62, but we mainly used to whinge to each other about anything and everything. We were well matched on that score. Steve lived in Walkington and I lived in the city, so we used to meet at South Cave, on the outskirts of Hull, every morning. He is a good bloke and we became very good friends.

It was quite a strange atmosphere at Belle Vue, but maybe it was understandable because the players they had the previous year had kept them in Super League. The likes of Gary Price and Andy Fisher had worked really hard the year before. I don't know whether there was a bit of resentment towards us newcomers, it just never gelled there. Wakefield was quite a cliquey club, and although the club tried to bring people in from other places, the existing players collectively made it difficult for us to settle and that was a big issue for me as soon as I got there.

Linzi never really enjoyed Wakefield. It was hard for her to settle in at the club, with the travelling. She worked full-time and only ever came across on game days; therefore she didn't really get to know anybody properly, with the exception of a couple of girls. We weren't very happy at the club especially as Hull had been such a friendly, sociable club. Any club we went to after that would have been hard pressed to follow. The attitude at Belle Vue was such a contrast to the one when I first joined Hull. Those players at the Boulevard felt it was great to sign myself and Huntey – and looked ahead to better things in the future, whereas at Wakefield I got the impression they thought they could do without us.

It was daunting – the other problem was that I didn't know anybody in the beginning. At least when I went to Hull, I knew both Huntey and Simon Booth. Even though I found it hard to settle and there was no real spirit, at the end of the day it was a job and I was grateful to them for giving me the opportunity.

Coaches Andy Kelly and his assistant Jon Sharp were good at what they did. They gave out new player booklets and had set moves and a game plan. Sharp impressed me as an assistant and I could see then he was going to be a good coach. He tried to improve individuals and that was the first bit of one to one coaching I had. He tried to look at my defence, because he must have seen that was the weakest part of my game. Although the coaching was okay, the real problem was the team not gelling.

Other clubs were doing pre-season training somewhere warm, but for Wakefield that year's camp was at Lincoln College. It was supposed to be a bonding exercise and we stayed in the dormitories. It was a good time, and they tried to get us doing team activities like canoeing and abseiling. On one of the nights at the student bar, there was a theme night 'leather and lace.' There was hardly anybody there and it was a bit of fun for students at the college. In that situation the worst thing anyone can do is ring home and tell someone that all the lads were going to a 'leather and lace' night. Although we were only in for an hour for a drink, one of lads told his wife what he was doing. The day after there was the biggest argument among all the lads. All you heard was, 'My wife's been on the phone ...' they were all going mad at each other. Basically as soon as one wife or girlfriend had been told, it spread like wildfire and the lads were all squirming. They had a meeting and people were trying to find out who had spilled the beans, so to speak. Maccer and I were laughing our heads off, because our wives were probably the only ones who had not been rung. It shows you what Chinese whispers can do and eventually one lad put his hand up and apologised. All the Wakey lads in the clique were fuming. Even though in all honesty it had been a rubbish night, the shit storm afterwards made it really funny.

Our first pre-season game was against Castleford on Boxing Day at Wheldon Road and we drew 14 all. We had a lot of youngsters playing but you could see there was real rivalry between the sides – which were both fired up just like a Saints v Wigan or Humberside derby game.

Our Challenge Cup run did not last long; we were hammered by Bradford in our second round with Bulls' Michael Withers scoring a hat-trick. Full back Withers impressed me as an opposite number. He is like a ghost and a really underestimated player in that great Bradford team. That defeat gave us a bit of wake up to what was coming that year.

We needed a kick up the arse for our next game at Leeds, knowing that the first game of the Super League season was going to be tough. It was a Friday night with local rivalry and everybody was up for it. I always seemed to play okay on Headingley's massive open pitch and I liked the atmosphere. My stats after the game showed that I had made 20 hit ups and 20 tackles, which is not bad for a full back. We were so switched on that we ended up winning so it was a great start to the Super League season.

Our form was patchy from then onwards, even though we beat a Warrington side featuring Alfie Langer. When we lost at home to London, coach Andy Kelly laid into us because he could see the pressure building up on him and was clutching at straws. I got a stinger in my shoulder in that game when I tackled someone from the scrum. My arm went dead and I really struggled with it for weeks after that. As a player you try and run injuries off so I strapped it up and played on. It affects your game and how you tackle, which wasn't one of my greatest attributes as it was, and I wasn't playing at my best.

After the promise of that first win, it was now a case of avoiding the drop, Andy Kelly and Jon Sharp were moved on and Tony Kemp and John Harbin took over as caretaker coaches. During their first training session, Kemp was quite clearly trying to motivate the team to finish the season off well. Harbin, who had been involved with the youngsters at the club, was very old school with outdated ideas and contributions to training sessions, which didn't go down well with the lads.

Later on when Tony Kemp resigned, with only a few games left, Harbin took over and then continued to coach them the following year. I was not the only one who felt that Harbin didn't know what he was doing but he seemed to be able to bullshit his way into jobs. The performances on the pitch were only part of the story – off it there were all kinds of drama going on which did not help our morale or performances.

Wakefield started off the season really positively and when they said they were trying to sign Jason Robinson and Jonah Lomu, we thought we were going places. Fast forward a few months and the cheques started bouncing. Investments never materialised and it brought the club to its knees really. They built the stand behind the sticks, but it became a symbol of the club's cack-handedness and looked like a block of Benidorm holiday flats. It was a grotesque attachment to a ground that had not changed much from when they filmed Richard Harris in *This Sporting Life* there in the early sixties. When it started going wrong, the club was left with no alternative but to put in for CVA. After one game they had to wait until the turnstile operators had cashed up to pay us our wages in fivers and pound coins. It was then that we knew the situation was dire.

The weeks when we did not get paid began to affect the team and we were called to a meeting in the poky little office at the back of the changing room. In that room we were basically told by a director that the club had no money and that they could not pay us. Scrum half Bobbie Goulding in particular was fuming and he barked at them, 'We have all got families, you are well out of order.' I thought he was going to smack him and as he stormed out of the door and slammed it as hard he could behind him, one of the polystyrene ceiling tiles fell down and just missed the director sitting below, which brought laughter to what otherwise was a very serious situation. It was a repeat of the previous year at Hull and made me think about whether rugby league was worth all the hassle. We got in touch with the GMB union but they were useless when we needed them and were powerless to do anything.

As it happened, I was shopping in Hull and bumped into Shaun McRae. I asked him in jest if he had a vacancy for a full back next year and if he was interested in me coming back. He told me he would have a word with Shane Richardson, chief executive, and that is all that was said. I don't know what happened but the shit really hit the fan afterwards, because people at Wakefield began to blank me and attitudes changed. Kemp and Harbin called me in for a meeting asking if I still wanted to play for the club. I said yes I did, not mentioning or even thinking about my conversation with 'Bomber', as it really was just in passing with no formality whatsoever. I had not spoken about contracts and my agent was not involved. But I knew there were money problems so I was trying to look after myself. What had I done wrong?

That week they told me I was dropped, then they changed their mind and I ended up playing on the wing with Paul Sampson at full back. I asked them to tell me if they had a problem with me on the field and told them they should not be dropping me over some sort of rumour. I am not sure how that innocent conversation got back to Wakefield, but I was able to work out the common denominator. The late David Topliss had connections with both clubs and he may not have realised he was getting me into trouble. It was something and nothing but Kemp fell out with me over that. All I was trying to do was plan ahead; after all I had been in this situation before. Two weeks later it all went belly up, as predicted.

The club went into CVA and that was it. The players' contracts were terminated for those of us aged over 24. Loads of players were sacked – Steve McNamara, Glen Tomlinson, Francis Maloney, Bobbie Goulding, Willie Poching, Warren Jowitt, Martin Masella and I were among those shown the door. We effectively ended up getting five weeks' sick pay and five weeks' holiday pay from the government. Once all this happened, I signed a two-year contract at Hull, but we still had to last until November without a wage. It was really annoying that 12 months later this had happened to me again. The lads took Wakefield to court for our wages but I did not even bother going because I knew CVA meant we would get balls all. We got something daft back, like £300, but it was only a token sum considering I had approximately £50k left to run on my contract. A lot of players lost out on big money with Wakefield's collapse.

They still had to pay for the stand behind the posts so players like us were not even the primary creditors. We were right near the bottom on the food chain but after all we had only played for the club and put our bodies on the line for the club. It was turmoil at the end but the season meant nothing to me. It would be difficult to say I enjoyed it. Rugby is rugby and you just do your job. I had signed for Wakefield for two years but part of me was just glad to get out after one. It was certainly an experience at Belle Vue, but it was even worse when I had to go back the following year as an opponent because their fans chanted, 'Judas!' and, 'You'll never get your money!' at me which was a bit harsh.

7

Ireland Calls

Although I had already represented England, Mick McGurn asked me if I had any Irish blood in my family. I did, under the grandparent ruling, and I jumped at the chance to play for Ireland. Mick phoned Ireland manager Steve O'Neill as they were starting to strengthen their squad. It was 1998 and I would play for Ireland along with the likes of Shaun Edwards, Gary Connolly, Chris Joynt and fantastic props, Terry O'Connor, Barry McDermott and Neil Harmon, as well as many other great players who I never would otherwise have had the opportunity to play alongside. I was enjoying my rugby at the time and playing internationally meant the world to me, especially with the high profile individuals in the team.

It was good to see what the Ireland management were trying to do. Steve O'Neill tried to bring in lads from the fledgling Irish competition, with players from Dublin Blues and Bangor Vikings given a go. They had not played at the highest of levels so understandably they didn't have the best skills. However, Steve also gave Brian Carney a chance and he ended up at Gateshead. It worked for him and then he went on to play for Great Britain, which is quite an achievement within a few years.

Steve also brought in three big name Aussies, Luke Ricketson, Kevin Campion and Danny Williams. There was a good feeling of camaraderie, that this was a squad coming together for the World Cup in 2000. When the Super League season ended the whole Irish squad got together with conditioner McGurn at Huddersfield and then we went for warm weather training at Club La Manga in Spain.

The facilities and training out there was superb. They gave us the first day off so me and Tommy Martyn went for a stroll around the massive five star training complex, but at midday we heard voices from a pub, 'Come in here and get on the lash with us.' We looked at each other and went in. It was a session but not of the training variety, the beer was flowing and we started playing drinking games. It turned into an all-dayer, which is probably not the best start to a training week! Alcohol changes people in different ways and I have met loads of rugby players who get really aggressive and want to fight after a few jars. It is opposite with me – when I get drunk I just want to have a laugh and muck about. But boy did I make myself look stupid that night after getting absolutely smashed. Looking back I can't believe that nobody from the management could see that and send me back to the hotel when it began to get out of control. Instead I was left to my own devices and ended up playing darts ... with a pool cue ... completely stark-bollock naked. Much of it is hazy, but the other lads were also as pissed as me and were messing around, swimming in the big fountain in the foyer of this impressive hotel. This was nothing to do with me, to my knowledge, I didn't get wet, but it was chaos as I made my way to bed.

Next morning came the aftermath. A really stony-faced Steve O'Neill entered the room after calling a team meeting. He ripped into us with the words, 'You're a set of bastards. They are going to throw us out of the hotel. It is going to be in the papers so I want to know who is responsible.' After putting my head down I could feel all eyes staring at me. Not just one or two, the whole team had turned towards me. I remember thinking, 'Surely it wasn't just me causing pandemonium last night?' But I thought I should face the music and said 'It was me, I'm responsible.'

Steve O'Neill was fuming with me and it was like I had taken a knife and had stuck it in to his back. He would not speak to me then and it bothered me that I had upset him so much. Although I have never walked away from anything in my life I was so upset then that I nearly did. The following night they made an example of me, making me dress up in a girl's outfit. It was not a good night for me because I had plenty on my mind and was so upset that I was close to quitting the squad, going home and not playing in the

World Cup. I felt alienated from the rest of the guys but Ireland's assistant coach Andy Kelly had a chat with me and explained that not everyone was upset with me and he persuaded me to stay. I was really grateful to him for that. In my defence I didn't cause a fight or any trouble, I just wanted to get some team-bonding going just like at Hull and Saints. I soon realised that it was more serious here and it gave me the impetus to do well and earn back the respect I lost that night. I didn't touch another drop until the tournament started.

When we went to Belfast, in preparation for the first game, the camaraderie returned and all the lads went to a pub where they had organised a band with songs, the drinks were flowing, but needless to say I didn't have a drink. There was a real attempt to Irish up the team; all the traditional songs and anthems were great. We bonded really well, embraced the culture, music and history in that great city. The heart and soul of the operation was my roommate, Martin Crompton, I woke him up every morning with the sounds of Irish music blasting out. He was a really nice bloke, a huge character and Irish through and through.

Although we had a quality team, we were still underdogs but won all three of our matches – against Samoa, Scotland and Maoris – in what was called the group of death. Our reward was England in the quarter finals, which we were happy with because we were on a roll. If we had finished second we would have played Australia, which I would have preferred. You want to play against the best to test yourself.

Prior to the game we made sure we sang with passion and looked at the opposition as we did. There was talk that England were vulnerable, especially with the quality of player Ireland had available. England were there for the taking, but I spent 10 minutes in the sin-bin after getting back to tackle Darren Rogers. He grabbed hold of me and I could not get off and so was sin binned straight away. Gutted by the call, I kept pacing the sidelines, hoping England wouldn't score while I was off the field, but inevitably they did and we lost 26-16.

Our team motto was 'spirit is our strength' and Terry O'Connor said it was the proudest moment of his career. We gave our loudest ever rendition of 'Ireland's Call' back in the dressing room and had a good drink afterwards, but I was fed up because we lost which meant this was the end. At first representing Ireland, for me, was just me wanting to play rugby, but it grew on me and I was passionate at the end. There was a feeling that we were playing for a cause, making Ireland big in rugby league and uniting the country by putting up a good show.

8

Back on Humberside

Hull FC was a different club to the bedraggled Hull Sharks outfit I had left in such turmoil just a year previously. At the helm, Shaun McRae was a successful coach and he brought a lot of Australians down from Gateshead with him after the two clubs had merged, and they complemented the good local Hull lads.

For all the changes, it was reassuring to see that there were still some of the old faces around at the Boulevard. The office staff, by and large, remained the same and a lot of the younger lads coming through had been kept on. Although former coach Steve Crooks was still there, he was now back in his original role, looking after the academy lads and there had been big changes at the top with Shaun McRae and Tony Anderson now the top men.

Tony was an impressive assistant coach, who studied rugby and more or less ran the show. That was Bomber's style – he was like that when he coached me at Saints too, where he delegated well to his assistant Mike Gregory. In Shane Richardson we had an authoritative chief executive in charge who most were frightened of and who was really tight with the purse strings. I guess that was what was needed after the last regime. He was the boss and we knew it. I got a taste of that from Richo early on. Before a ball had been kicked Tony Grimaldi, Luke Felsch and I were nominated to go in to negotiate Challenge Cup money. I was now classed as a senior player and this procedure is normal practice at most clubs. The CEO just would not budge, which was not the normal outcome. There was no negotiation, it was a take it or leave it conversation.

When I was playing at Wakefield, I remembered one of sponsors threw something into the Challenge Cup pot as an incentive, so I had the temerity to mention that in our negotiations with Richo. Well he hit the roof and walked all over us saying, 'Look, there are academy players fighting for places and you lot want more money!' The others were cowering and I felt an inch tall. The other guys never said as much as a squeak. When we got out Grimo and Felschy laughed at me for trying it on when they could see it was a losing battle. I did it for all the boys as I felt I owed it to them for nominating me and I wanted to try my best. I quickly named them 'Zippy' to the boys when we had to go back with the bad news. I knew from that meeting that I would never be on 'The Apprentice' but at least I can say I tried.

It was quite a good atmosphere at Hull FC and although two clubs had merged there were no Hull/Gateshead club cliques. All the Aussie players, their wives and girlfriends were friendly and as a group we socialised. Team wise we had quality with hooker Lee Jackson returning from his stint in Australia, and two great halves in Tony and Jason Smith, complementing the young Richard Horne and Paul Cooke.

It was wonderful to go back to Hull – no more travelling and a great calibre of players. I felt like I was back home, even though Hull was my adopted city. It just felt right. Hull had a good team – a big pack and plenty of craft at half back. For me, though, it was all about scoring tries and so running off the halves like Jason Smith, who could create a hole in the defence from nothing, was good for my game.

We also found out why Jason was nicknamed Animal on the pre-season trip to Lanzarote. The whole week away was hilarious and it was the first time I had been away properly for warm weather training. Jason had just signed, and he created quite a first impression. On our first day they gave us free rein to have a beer. We met up with the London Broncos boys who were over there too. Jason knew a lot of the Aussie Broncos and ended up getting wrecked with them. He was well away, dancing to a song when he fell over and smashed his head before coming up with the biggest gash I have ever seen, with blood pumping out everywhere. I managed to stem the flow with a beer towel but, because of state he was in, he started blaming me. Tony Grimaldi and I took him to the medical centre. He was completely blasé about the blood pouring out and was swearing his head off and cursing the doctors so much so I don't think the medical staff gave him anaesthetic when they stitched him up.

The next morning Billy Mallinson took over the training session at the sports centre and he put us on the line and had us doing 100 metre turnarounds. We had to do 10 of them in 14 seconds or less. We set off and Jason Smith was just trotting along, still feeling the effects of the night before, 20 metres behind the rest of us. Bomber would just say, 'Billy, add another one on!' This was funny at first, but by the fourth extra one the lads became irritated and began shouting and swearing out loud. Shaun obviously knew what we were going through, especially Jason, so just thought he would add to the pain but Billy could see our frustration and adjusted the timings in our favour. It gave us a warning that Bomber could still be hard.

The real joker in the pack was Tony Smith, who we called Casper, and he took the piss out of everyone, especially Lee 'Jacko' Jackson and me in that first year. Casper is funny – if difficult – because it was hard to get your own back on him as he was so quick witted you knew you wouldn't win. I was amused by this and didn't take it to heart but I am sure he upset a few people.

We meant business that year, and it was a measure on how far Hull had come when we rocked Saints to the core in our next fixture, only narrowly losing our unbeaten record 38-34.

A few games into the season and it had become really clear that Jason Smith had really got hold of this team. Jason was the best player I have played with – a different type of ball player to Bobbie Goulding and Tommy Martyn, who I had played with at Saints. Jason played like a rough forward and could tackle, knock them off and yet he had the soft hands of a ball player. He was a complete rugby player.

One of the highlights of that year for me was the really close game at Halifax, which was 28-all with one minute to go. We worked up the field from deep in our half and both Jason Smith and Tony Smith were weighing up a drop goal. As everybody looked at each other, I said, 'I'll have it.' From 46 yards out I hit the ball – one of the worst connections of a drop kick I can recall – but it just kept going. When it went over I just ran towards the Hull fans that were going absolutely crazy in the away end. Chief executive Shane Richardson came bounding across the pitch and made a beeline for me and was jumping on me saying how brilliant it was.

We won eight of our last nine games to finish third, but it is what we deserved because we were up there for a good part of the year.

As the third placed side we travelled to Wigan in our first play-off game, but were devastated by injuries to two key players and narrowly went down 27-24. Jason Smith dislocated an elbow and Tony Smith went off and I can seriously say, had both Smiths played in the second half, it may have been different. We had another bite of the cherry, a home eliminator against Saints. The packed Boulevard was in full voice that night, but the luck was with Saints and we were pipped 20-24. Hull competed with the big boys that year for the first time in a long time, but we could not quite finish it off in the crunch, must-win games to get to the Grand Final. It was a good experience for the young lads, Paul Cooke, Richard Horne and Paul King, but maybe inexperience took its toll in the end. To cap a good season I won the player of the year award at the end of season ceremony, which was unbelievable given the calibre of individual talent I played alongside.

Everybody at Hull was keen to build on what we had achieved in 2001 and a declaration that we meant business was the fact that we returned to Lanzarote for our warm weather pre-season training. It made for an interesting week, staying 10 to a villa and with there being so many lads in one room, pranks were a plenty. Logan Campbell and I were in our element and we decided that Andy Last and Craig Poucher would be the perfect 'couple' for our entertainment. Pouch had been ill leading up to the trip and so he had an early night whilst the rest of us went out. We returned before the others and found an onion in the kitchen, finely chopped it and stuffed it in Lasty's pillow. When Lasty came back to the room, he immediately acknowledged the aroma, and Craig woke up and was overly apologetic; truly believing it was his body odour that was to blame for the smell. Being such a nice guy that Lasty is, he just accepted it and got his head down to get some sleep. However, during the middle of the night we were woken by a bemused Andy Last who entered our room and proceeded to empty the contents of the stinking pillow case over myself and Logan. The next morning we were all tickled by the fact that Craig Poucher believed that his arm pits could actually smell so bad.

There were a few incidents, not all of them as light-hearted as Oniongate. Big, bruising Aussie prop forward Craig Greenhill had come to the club to replace Paul Broadbent. Well the big fella was called Knuckles and we soon discovered why. He kept winding Gareth Raynor up in Lanzarote by calling him a derogatory name that finally provoked a reaction. One night I was woken up by a hell of a commotion after Gaz Raynor had eventually flipped and had flown at Knuckles which was not the best of moves. Gaz threw a glass, which ended up hitting one of the unlucky peacemakers, cutting his head. I jumped up and with a couple of other lads got in between them but then immediately thought, 'What the hell am I doing here?' Knuckles' big fist was clunking me on the back of the head as he tried to get his punches in on Gaz. So I let go, and they were really going at it hammer and tongs. You could hear the blows connecting, it was pretty brutal stuff and Knuckles smashed Gaz through the patio window before picking him up and punching him again. Me and the other lads jumped in at that point and managed to part them.

It was just boys letting off steam; a little bit of name calling that had gone too far. The players offered to pay for the windows and explained that it was an 'accident'. As a team bonding exercise it was probably a little extreme that night because it was more like a war zone. Imagine the scene the following morning – a baking hot day in Lanzarote – Gaz came to training wearing a woolly hat to hide his battle scars. It was definitely no holiday camp and we trained three times a day – fieldwork in the morning and early evening and weights in the afternoon.

Our team bonding continued when we returned to Humberside and we went out round Hull with new signing Graham Mackay for the first time. As we went into one pub the DJ announced, 'Look here's the Adams Family, look at Uncle Fester!' referring to Mackay who had a bald head. Mackay, who was 6ft 5 and built like a brick outhouse, took exception and threw a glass ashtray in the DJ's direction and it smashed, sending glass everywhere.

My good friend Logan Campbell and I thought it would be funny to ask the DJ in the next pub we went in to tell everyone that Uncle Fester was in. We knew there may be a consequence so to make it fair, we did rock paper scissors to see which one of us would ask. Unfortunately, I lost, so had to do the asking but didn't spot Graham stood right behind me. Within ten minutes he had me upside down and was drilling my head into the couch. We thought it was a laugh, but after seeing the look on his face he didn't find it at all funny. It is fair to say I kept my distance from him after that.

That was not the worst misfortune that befell me that season and in July I suffered from a dreadful ailment called labyrinthitis, which came on me suddenly at training. Driving home I had to get out of my car because the illness affected my balance and made me heave. It felt like I was going to fall down and when I got home and went to bed I could not lift my head off the pillow. Stupidly, during recovery, I played against Saints which was a nightmare because every time the ball went up into air I could not see it. It was one of those things you do as a pro – play on because you think you're okay, but there was no way I should have been out there. My eyes were not focusing at all, so when Craig Greenhill made a break, I supported him but could not see the ball as he passed it to me and so I dropped it. Needless to say I was taken off shortly after.

Hull coach Shaun McRae had become a lot more professional, although in my opinion I thought he could have done more on the training field and help to improve weaknesses. Despite being the boss, one particular week he found himself the butt of the jokes. At Hull the lads had a thing called 'goose of the week.' Basically, at the pre-match meal, once a week we would talk about any funny things that the lads had done in the preceding seven days – and the worst culprit was nominated 'goose of the week' and had to wear the t-shirt. The shirt was not allowed to be washed and the victims had to sign it, so you can imagine the disgusting state of it. It was all a bit of fun at the end of a hard week of training.

So when we were all sat around the table discussing 'goose of the week', I urged Deon Bird to tell a story that he had told me earlier in the week. He was a little reluctant at first but all the boys encouraged him and he gave in, but it may have unintentionally ended up getting him in lumber. Deon said, 'When I went to the toilet earlier in the week, Bomber came in and stood at the next urinal. I couldn't believe it when he pulled his tracksuit bottoms and underpants down, round his ankles, while he had a pee. I've not done that since I was five.' Everyone was laughing and as a result Shaun was given the 'goose of the week' shirt. To his credit, he accepted it and wore the smelly shirt for the training session. It may be completely unrelated, but two weeks later Birdy was sold to Castleford after being released from his contract. Every time Birdy's wife, Sarah saw me afterwards she always joked with me that I had got her husband sacked.

During the course of the season the former England coach, John Kear, came in as an assistant coach and we went back to basics. We began working on core skills again which was a breath of fresh air and Kear was really good for us and I enjoyed learning and working under him. It really reinvigorated me. John's presence and input was a good change for Hull and most of the lads agreed. It was good to learn and watch things develop, and the key seemed to be trying to get quicker play the balls. Again we made the play-offs and our last competitive game was our knockout by Leeds. The Rhinos had the game sewn up with four minutes left when our mischievous hooker Lee Jackson worked a bit of Tommy Cooper style magic. We had won a penalty, which we kicked to touch, but Jacko had already sneaked the spare ball up the back of his jersey. He quickly tapped it from the mark and touched down while everyone else stood still waiting for the ball to come back from the ball boy. The Leeds players did not lay a finger on him – and their coach Daryl Powell was fuming afterwards because they gave the try. Ref Russell Smith was baffled by the furore and consulted his touch judge, and then it went to the video referee, who had not spotted what Jacko had done and awarded the try.

That was not the end of the year – we had the important matter of saying goodbye to the Boulevard with a finale against the touring Kiwis. It was supposed to be a memorable occasion in front of one final packed house at the famous old ground. Unfortunately, it only lasted 10 minutes for me. After taking a pass out the back from a scrum I tipped it on and then relaxed. Thud! A big Kiwi forward had connected at full speed and I hit the deck with a grade three rupture of my AC joint. My arm was knackered and I could not move it. Our physio came on the pitch and said, 'If you come off, you won't be able to go back on!' It shocked me a little because I thought I would have been automatically off because my shoulder was a mess. 'He must think I'm okay,' I thought to myself so tried to carry on despite the agony. We scored from that passage of play, but inevitably the Kiwis' kick off came straight to me. After catching it I went to pass it, but my shoulder seemed to separate from my body so I immediately put my good arm up and told them to get me off.

It was one of the worst injuries I have had but the specialist said I could leave it and let it heal itself or have it operated on. He assured me that the recovery time would be exactly the same for either option. I let it heal itself. If I knew what I know now, I would have chosen the other option. My shoulder is disfigured and I have been left with a large bulge on my left side, which is often commented on when I take my top off or wear a vest at the gym or on holiday. The injury caused me problems in 2003, particularly with tackling. To be honest, my shoulder was knackered after that which meant I always had to wear a protective cover over it and it was touch and go whether it would be approved by the laws of the game. The touch judges used to come into the dressing room to check us over before we went out, so I would put my protection mould on to my shoulder and then pad it up and strap it on.

With the exception of my shoulder injury, 2003 was a good year for me; I was probably playing the best rugby of my career. I felt I had matured physically and felt strong mentally too. It was also a good year for the club because we had moved out of the Boulevard to a brand new KC Stadium. The new pitch was 67 metres wide, which suited my style of rugby down to the ground. KC is a great stadium to play in and the atmosphere was always so good and alive.

Our first home league game was built up as 'the big one' to officially mark our new ground and we were expected to put in a good performance. Unfortunately, the event was a real damp squib and we just could not score against a tough-tackling London Broncos. However, we went well in the league and there was a growing feeling of optimism after we beat Wigan 20-4 at home. Our league game at Headingley was a real classic in which we were better in the first half and Leeds were in charge for the second half. We trailed by two points when we were awarded a dubious late penalty by referee Steve Ganson for offside. There were literally no seconds on the clock so all the players were saying, 'Two points.' I walked over slowly and tried to get myself together. All of a sudden Leeds' big prop Ryan Bailey appeared in front of me trying to put me off. I said to the ref, 'Have a word with this guy!' but then big Barrie Mac started doing the same thing and even Rob Burrow was waving his arms. I just concentrated on where I was going to aim and I knew from all the hours of practice, how much movement I got from each kick. It was a matter of lining the ball up correctly on the tee. I knew I could do it but I have got to say I did feel the pressure. I struck it beautifully and it sailed over. Seeing all the Hull fans in background reacting to it like we had won the league, made me realise how much it meant to these loyal away supporters.

My confidence was sky high at this point; I was scoring a lot of points and even earned the Super League Player of the Month award. So when we played Saints I was determined to have a good game with it being my home town club. People still remind me of this game and seem to call it 'the Darren Albert game.' This was my best ever performance against Saints. Albert was the quickest in the league and had won a sprint competition earlier that season but I scored a great try, outfoxing him on the way. Although the Aussie speedster caught me, I had the experience to move my body to one side, like Ellery Hanley used to do, and that left Albert trailing. To cap it off I then did a trademark big dive in front of the Saints fans. I think the emotion of scoring against my old club got the better of me that day. It was a great feeling.

I continued scoring points and at one spell I held the record for the top try scorer and top points scorer in the league. I scored a brace of tries and kicked six goals in the hammering of my former club, Wakefield, at the KC Stadium on June 26. It would not have been worthy of such a note except they would turn out to be my last points in my final game for Hull FC. Obviously I did not know what was around the corner.

9

Career Break

My dad had played for Lancashire in the seventies and earned his county cap, which was an achievement I always wanted to emulate. When I was growing up we had a trophy cabinet in our dining room where all my dad's honours took pride of place. As I grew older, I used to ask my dad to tell me what each award was for and the red velvet Lancashire cap was always one of my favourites. So when coach Paul Cullen picked me to play in Lancashire's Origin game against Yorkshire, I was delighted. Some players probably viewed it as a 'nothing game' and had enough of representative rugby but I really wanted to play and get one of those red caps of my own. It was on my mind that I was carrying a calf strain, but I wasn't going to let that stop me. I was looking forward to playing, especially as I would be teaming up with old friends Scully, Keiron Cunningham and Longy at a representative level.

The game wasn't what I had expected and the performance from Lancashire was below par. Yorkshire stand-off, Chris Thorman, was outstanding and their team really performed, making it a very one sided game.

Niggling injuries meant I came off the bench but tried to get stuck in and make an immediate impression. The fateful moment of the match for me came when ex-Wakefield team-mate and Yorkshire loose forward Ryan Hudson broke straight through. I knew I would have to get him down, to eliminate him from the next play so I went in hard. The force of the collision between my right knee and his had disastrous consequences and I remember being on the floor thinking, 'Something isn't right.' As I tried to get to my feet and move on the spot, my leg felt weird and within seconds I was in agony, put my hand up and they carried me off.

Chris Brookes, the Wigan doctor, came in to see me in the dressing room and his first diagnosis was a dislocated kneecap. He gave me some pain relief, strapped it up and handed me some crutches. After seeing Linzi, I called Hull's physio who told me not to go to A & E, but to travel back to Humberside and wait until the morning when he would organise a private consultation. If I had gone to the local infirmary they would have probably put my leg in plaster rather than a brace, hindering my recovery.

My knee was throbbing all night and I did not sleep a wink. It was x-rayed the following day and after they had syringed 110ml of blood out of it they said it was good news – I had fractured my knee! The bottom of my patella had been split off, but apparently, that was better than a dislocation, which would have the additional complication of ligament damage.

The first prognosis with the fracture was six to ten weeks on the sidelines so I still had high hopes of returning before the end of the year. I endured a daily session of physio with Keith Warner, who was known to the lads as Cheggers because he looked so much like BBC presenter Keith Chegwin. He tried hard to get me back, and had me doing a lot of cycling and leg strengthening exercises. In August we cycled from Hull to Withernsea on the most clapped-out bikes I had ever seen. We basically rode 30 miles to the coast, had fish and chips for dinner and then cycled back. The bikes were so awful that afterwards I thought to myself, 'I'm not going through that again'. I thought ahead and spoke to my club sponsor Mark Jackson from KG Engineering in Hull, fortunately he loaned me his beautiful, lightweight bike with great handlebars. It was worth £2,500 and I was most appreciative. It was a dream to ride, so the next time we went out I raced to Withernsea leaving poor Richard Fletcher on his clapped-out old bike half an hour behind me. In future years, when I started to do the cycling challenges, I made sure I had a good carbon bike to make the difficult challenges that little bit less gruelling.

The time went on in rehab but I still had weakness and strange pains when exercising and an odd clicking sound when I straightened my knee. As the season came to a close I began to question if the rehabilitation plan was the right one for me so went to see the specialist again and he advised me to have an operation, under general anaesthetic, whilst they explored whether I had a bone spur which could have been hindering my recovery.

During the weeks leading up to Christmas, I went for surgery. When I came out the day after the arthroscopy and shaving, I was told that the bone spur was fine, but there was slight damage to the cartilage that had been fixed and he had done a bit of cleaning up around the tendon on the bone. The surgeon's report stated, 'I arthroscoped knee and surprisingly found a little lateral meniscus tear, which I trimmed and debraded the patellar tendon in section. His symptoms will settle, but I think his recovery will be rather prolonged.' If he thought there was nothing wrong, why did his report state that it would be a prolonged recovery?

In January the report said he 'saw no purpose of further intervention and has no plans to see me.'

Hull's new physio Simon Pope joined in January 2004 and six months on from the initial injury I was still struggling. In the meantime new players were coming in and I was still kicking my heels on the sidelines. I was desperate to train and did a bit of boxing, but could not really join in any of the other exercises because my knee was so sore. During the player appraisal in the off-season, I asked what I needed to do to get back on the pitch. The pressure to play was intensifying now, I felt pushed out of the squad and little remarks, which were funny at first, began to grate on me, comments such as 'here come the patio club' when the injured players came on to the field. It wasn't the players making the remarks but the coaching staff. It made me feel like they didn't appreciate the hard work I was putting in. I was battling in desperation to get back playing for the club, yet as the time went on it seemed that the staff had forgotten about my ability on the field and made me the butt of their jokes. People's attitudes were changing.

All I wanted was to feel part of the squad, but I was continuing to train separately and so no longer felt part of the team. During the close season, they recruited and, amongst others, brought in talented young full back Shaun Briscoe from Wigan ahead of the 2004 season. John Kear had coached Shaun previously at Wigan and I felt he wanted him to be Hull's number one. I could understand the reasoning behind it, with me struggling to regain full fitness.

Brisc was, and still is, a great lad who came in with a completely different attitude to what I had done in my early days at Saints with Dave Lyon. It was like a roles reversal and this time it was my number one jersey up for grabs. I took to Shaun straight away, with no resentment whatsoever, but still in my mind I wanted to get back on the pitch and get my career back on track.

I suppose the frustrating situation made me feel like a piece of meat, but rugby league is a business. According to the terms, Hull were within their rights to terminate my contract because I had been out for more than six months. The club did not push this at first, they gave me more time, but they did tell me that it had been discussed. This was then planted in my mind and the pressure was now on me and the club's physio to get me right. Simon Pope was a former football physio and he worked the living daylights out of me, which made me even more determined to get back. Although I was no expert, I told Simon I needed to start running but he said I needed to build up the quads and stabilisers around my knee first.

The 'more time' that I had been initially given didn't last that long. On February 6 I was called to a meeting with Hull FC chief executive Dave Plummer where I was basically given six to twelve weeks to prove my fitness. The club were getting tired of waiting for my return to the pitch so I decided that I needed to go for it. It may have been my imagination but I told the physio that my leg was now feeling strong. Maybe I was being positive and saying 'go for it' because I was so desperate to play. At the end of February we went to Leeds United's training ground and did a few different things, stuff that I was not doing in the gym with monotonous regularity. It involved a bit more movement and I even did some running on the trampoline. It gave me a taste for running again and in my physio notes stated, 'I wanted to run, but the physio was not letting me.' By early March I was allowed to run properly for the first time on a treadmill. My tendon was well strapped and I started to notice the effect of the tape easing the pain.

The physio decided to send me for an ultrasound scan on my knee with a consultant musculoskeletal radiologist. Then things became a little clearer – but not for the better. The results both shocked and angered me. A note back to the physio revealed, 'At the site of the patient's focal tendon abnormality there is a hypoechoic cleft present in the lateral portion of the patellar tendon. This correlates well with symptoms with a thin hypoechoic tract extending down to the joint space through Hoffa's fat pad ...' Basically, it was explained to me that I had a hole in my patellar tendon, one that had been most likely caused during the procedure by the previous surgeon in December.

I was so angry and two days later an MRI scan confirmed, 'A defect present in the lateral aspect of the patellar tendon.' It went on to read, 'The appearances are highly suggestive of change secondary to an arthroscopy portal having passed through the lateral aspect of the patellar tendon.'

I was gutted and fuming with what had been revealed. The notes clearly suggested that the surgeon had gone through my patellar tendon and left a hole in it. Then it all made sense – I had busted my balls to get back and now I realised my knee was not recovering because there was a hole in it. My head was in bits because by this stage it was eight months since I last played.

On March 19 I had a meeting with the physio, coach Shaun McRae and chief executive Dave Plummer to discuss the results and my options. That was followed by a further meeting with the solicitors where we discussed the case against the surgeon and raised the question of pay-outs in the event of me retiring. I made a legal statement which set out, step by step, what had happened to me from the night of the injury and subsequent treatment.

Hull kindly offered to start the proceedings and fund the fees up to a certain amount to see if we had a case. A further meeting with Plummer took place in April and by that stage I was doing a lot of work outside on the training pitch. I told him that I was a lot better training outside because I was stale inside and I was desperate to be involved with the team.

Ten days later I went to see the GMB union along with Plummer to see what they could do. Sadly, and not for the first time, it was not a lot. Back on the paddock I had started doing pulley sessions and I was pulling weights and in May I joined in the first team session. Although I was still limited to what I could do, I was back where I wanted to be. Much of my task was being stand in for Richard Swain as a hooker during the drills but I was delighted to be able to do this. However, at this stage the hierarchy at Hull must have had discussions about what would happen if I got injured in training and they put the brakes on what I was doing. After another limbo period we were now in to June and time had gone too far. We had another meeting with Plummer. I did not make a decision to quit; I was more or less forced to accept a six month notice period. It was classed as retiring, which dressed it up much nicer, but really they were giving me six months notice. I received a pay-off to walk away with but at the end of day I was out of a job – they had given me six months wages, yet I still had another 18 month contract left.

This was a junction in my life; I was only 30 and not ready to retire. It was nagging at the back of my head that I could have played on if things had been different. The question was 'Do I work my bollocks off and get back in as a professional at that age or find a new career?' How long did I have left as a professional? It came to a point and a realisation that my career was over. It was a really hard decision and I still think of it now, even with all I have been through with my illness, because rugby was my life. Rugby was in my blood and to give it up in that way was tough.

Previously, I had it in my head to play until I was 35. My dad played in the pack as a pro until he was 41 – and he was working too. That said, he is knackered now – his knees have gone, he has a bad shoulder and a sore neck. I did not want that to be like that, but full back was not as brutal as playing in the pack in the seventies and eighties. About a month after the retirement announcement was made, I was invited by Hull FC to lead the teams out at the KC Stadium to say my farewells to the crowd. Fittingly, it was against Saints on July 17 and I took my son Taylor out to the centre spot with me. Going out there was an extremely emotional experience. Although I walked out no problem, I could see all the Saints lads and crowd applauding too. Then I could see Hull hooker Richard Swain, who had tears in his eyes, which made me emotional. All the lads came over to give me a hug rather than a handshake. The tears were rolling down my face but I did not want to show it to my little boy Taylor. It made me sad to think that although he had been a part of rugby league and the great club Hull FC, who he loved, he would probably not remember watching me play the game and would not be a part of it anymore.

It was a loud KC Stadium send off and Hull won easily 34-6 that day.

That was that done with, but there was the important matter of getting my knee sorted out and apportioning blame as to why a supposedly straightforward injury had ended my career. When I finished playing I asked the Hull physio whether I could carry on attending because they had dealt with my problem. Popey said he did not see a problem with that. Then he checked with Hull FC and they said that it was not possible. It felt like they had washed their hands of me.

I went to see Gary Slade, my old physio at Wakefield and asked for a second opinion. He told me if I left the injury it would get worse. So that is when I decided to get it sorted out and went to see a consultant. At our first meeting he actually said he could feel a hole in my knee where the previous surgeon had gone through. That is when he said, 'I would not have done that.' At that time I asked Plummer if Hull FC would pay the costs to get my knee put right. They offered for so many physio sessions and then a consultancy, but they generously agreed to pay the full amount for the surgery as well. I was very grateful to them for doing that, but I was not sure if it was just to get me out of their hair or if they felt obliged to help me.

As for the legal case, we went to see a consultant orthopaedic surgeon in Manchester who looked at all the evidence around my knee. The club's solicitors were in charge of the case for me and Hull and they enlisted a surgeon to see if it was worth pursuing. The consultant wrote his report and basically, in his opinion, said it would probably be too hard to prove and too costly. This information was relayed to the solicitors and it was decided that the case against the surgeon would be closed.

I could never have imagined how hard it could be to give up something that is your life. It was a mentally tough time. I was worried about the financial aspect, supporting my family and continuing to live as we had done previously. We had to take a step back and reassess. Linzi had given up work to look after Taylor, so essentially we had no income. We knew the payout would not last forever and it was now time for me to make some changes in my life. But what should I do?

We still socialised with the families from the club. They were our friends and were always going to stay that way, but as time moves on you start to see less and less of everybody as your life begins to move away from rugby. I found it hard going from being in a team environment, which I had been a part of for my entire career. Work colleagues become like family members as you spend so much time together and you trust and rely on each other. You almost go through a battle together on the field and you form a strong bond. When that is taken away, it is a struggle to deal with mentally. I had no direction, no real qualifications and didn't know where I was heading. With no professional support network available, my family and I were left to get on with it. Since going through that, I have continued to encourage players to have something to fall back on after rugby. Rugby cannot last forever and whether it is your decision to retire or you are forced to retire, it is not easy.

It was time to move on – but I did not sever my links with Hull FC. The year after I retired Hull FC made it through to the Challenge Cup Final at the Millennium Stadium, Cardiff. Attending the game was a strange experience on a couple of levels. The match took place just after Linzi and I had returned from honeymoon after finally getting married. We travelled down early in the morning, taking Taylor with us. We were all shattered after a long flight back from Mauritius, but we wanted to be there to share the experience with Hull FC and our close friends who were still part of the team. We were sat next to probably the roughest family ever. The mother and father had about five teeth between them, even though they had kids with them, they effed and blinded all the way through. With Taylor, who was almost four, being with us we cringed the whole way through as we were not used to him hearing that sort of language.

At half time another couple sat in front of me, turned around and asked me for my autograph, but then I heard the dad from 'the family' say to his lad, 'Go and get that fella's autograph'. The lad took the signed piece of paper away and then after about 15 minutes of studying the signature the dad – a Hull fan – tapped me on the shoulder, and said, 'Go on then, I give up, who are you then?' Well Linzi and I began to laugh and that alone made the journey worthwhile.

Hull won the game with a late Paul Cooke try, converted by Danny Brough, which was a bit of a shock as Leeds were favourites. After the game we proudly watched the lads do a lap of honour and I was so pleased for them. I went down to the front and Chris Chester, Garreth Carvell and Kirk Yeaman spotted me and went out of their way to come over for a chat. It was nice that they acknowledged me at a time when they could have just gone on to celebrate their win.

It was nevertheless a difficult experience knowing that I could have been out there too. I wished I too could have joined in with the celebrations and been a part of the club winning some silverware. It felt like I had played a part in the rebuilding of Hull FC and loved the club and wanted it to be successful, but I would have given anything to have still been there at that time. But that is rugby and life – just look at my replacement Shaun Briscoe, who did not play in that game having been taken to hospital that week with appendicitis. He, too, must have shared in my mixed feelings of disappointment and elation.

10

Life After League

As for my own future outside of rugby, I had started to think about things the year before my injury and went back to college to get my GCSE mathematics. I was 29-30 then and you can't play rugby all your life. When you are playing and it is all going well you put it at the back of your mind and think you have everything. That is why I feel sorry for some of the lads now. They will think that rugby is going to secure their futures. I know there's a lot of money in the game and some might not have to worry unduly about their lives after rugby, but some will. Looking back I would have prepared earlier for the transition to life after rugby, but that is hindsight. That is one piece of advice I would offer to all young players today.

Clubs are now thinking more about their players – not just about the rugby aspect – particularly about looking after them in different ways. In my last year at Hull I did a rugby league Level 3 Coaching course, as all I could ever see myself doing was something within the game and I felt coaching was an option.

Just after I had retired from the game, Hull invited me to the Player of the Year awards where coach Shaun McRae made a presentation to celebrate my time with the team. It was a very emotional moment, in front of lots of people. I felt honoured to be there and the kind gesture showed their appreciation of the dedication and efforts I had given throughout my time at Hull. Mick Cox, the Head of Hull College Sports Department introduced himself to me and asked me whether I had thought about a career in teaching sport. This hadn't crossed my mind but the prospect sounded very appealing. After a lengthy conversation he mentioned that there may be an opportunity for a part-time post at the college. He told me to give him a ring and arrange to meet him later in the week to discuss it further. For the next few days my head was all over the place. I loved the thought of passing on my skills to young sports enthusiasts but on the other hand I questioned whether I had the ability to do so. I thought lots about it and talked it over with Linzi for hours and hours and finally plucked up the courage to give Mick a call and let him be the one to say whether I would be suitable. I went in for my first formal interview a nervous wreck, but I must have given the right answers as they offered me the job. Either that or they were desperate.

I was effectively a teaching assistant initially. I was teamed up with Stuart Horsfield – a really nice guy and a great teacher too. He had gone through the university route to become a sports teacher, but had no professional sporting experience, which is why I think it worked so well. It was a new course so the curriculum was new to both of us, which allowed us to have our own input and ideas. Level 1 Sport began with 18 students in its first year.

The first day in my new job was scary because I was going into another environment, one I never thought I would experience. Rugby had been my life, but I loved it from the start and it helped that I was with another member of staff who I gelled with straight away. I did feel inferior to the other teachers in the beginning because I had come into this from a different route. The majority of them helped me get over this and realise that my experience was invaluable in other ways and this helped me a lot, but it frightened me that I didn't have that teaching knowledge and the literacy skills. From the start the kids really respected me and I think that because I had only just finished playing was a big advantage. That year was absolutely brilliant. Together Stuart and I had some great ideas and made the course really enjoyable for the students and ourselves. It was great having the freedom to develop it from scratch. As things went on, I picked up more confidence and took the classes if Stuart was off. I did my City and Guilds 7307 teaching qualification one night a week. This enabled me to teach 16-19 year olds and the following year I started to do my Cert Ed, but circumstances with my health prevented me from completing the full qualification.

The paperwork was a bit of a problem at first, although Linzi helped me initially, and I brought a lot of work home. I wanted the kids to enjoy it and I think they did. We organised interesting events for the students which included spending a morning with Hull City FC, watching them train and analysing the coaching techniques and interviewing the coach, Peter Taylor, which they loved. We also arranged for guest speakers to come in and talk to the students and answer any questions they had. Although these were interesting and beneficial, not all were a success.

One morning, the Head of the Sports College arranged for a professional golfer to speak to the class. It was all done very quickly and unfortunately we failed to pick up his first name. All we knew was that it was a golfer called 'Finch' currently on the European Tour. The only golfer we could think of was Ian Baker Finch who had retired some years ago, so we were pretty sure it wasn't going to be him. When he arrived I was sent to greet him and he introduced himself as Richard Finch. I passed this information on to Stuart, but I had a smirk on my face and he was reluctant to believe me due to our good working relationship where we could have a laugh and wind each other up. When it came to introducing him to the class it was obviously Stuart's place to do so, but because of his uncertainty of his name he was nodding at me to do it and I was nodding back at him. So Stuart, covering his back and saving himself from any embarrassment, introduced him as 'The Golfer'. I nearly pissed myself. To him we must have looked totally unprofessional. Richard Finch is a name that will stay with me and still makes me chuckle.

Being a former player, the college asked me to help with the rugby league team. It was a good set up and Mark Brown a fellow colleague was the coach. We had a good first season and got to the cup final at Dewsbury coincidentally, against St Helens College, my home town. We were lucky enough to be able to select a few Academy players from Hull KR and Hull FC, due to the close relationship with the clubs, as the college had linked up and was educating the youngsters. We went on to win the cup and, considering we had one sent off before half time, we did really well and it was fantastic for the College and those who had coached the team.

While I was at Hull College, Richard Crompton, one of the members of staff, was involved at Hull Ionians. This got me thinking and talking about getting into rugby union. Rich invited me to go down to Ionians in the summer, so that I could join in the training. I wasn't nervous about the training itself, more about fitting in, and not being accepted socially with my league background. I also had concerns about not doing the right thing on the field as I wasn't up to speed with the rugby union rules. Ionians are based at Brantingham Park on the outskirts of Hull. So I went down and trained with them – and scored a few tries. I think the lads got a buzz out of it that year because I had joined them after just finishing with Hull FC, so it was seen to be a big capture for the club. It was both interesting and difficult at times. When you think of rugby union you think about the rucks and getting caught up in them but your adrenaline is flowing and you don't feel the stampings ... not until after the game anyway.

One game I came across an old acquaintance from my Great Britain rugby league days – John Bentley, who was coach of Cleckheaton. Bentos was giving out some real verbal stick to our fly-half, who had played for him the year before. Bentley kept shouting, 'Give it to him ... he'll bottle it.' I remember coming out for the second half and he shouted, 'You might as well be sitting with me Precky!' which was typical of him. Bentos is a nice guy, but always looking for ways to put you off your game.

My rugby union career nearly took another turn, courtesy of Brad Hepi, who was my team-mate for a spell at Hull. I was in my second year of teaching when Brad was taken on at the College. Brad told me that he was going on the England Rugby Union Veterans' tour to Durban in South Africa and asked if I wanted to go. He asked me to play in Terry Fanalua's testimonial at Kingsholm, Gloucester and I scored a 50 metre try going around wing Marcel Garvey in the process and getting a big cheer from the Gloucester rugby union fans. They must have thought I was a half-decent player by this time. The coach on the sidelines nudged Brad and said, 'He's coming to South Africa with us.' It was all sorted and then after thinking about it, I realised it probably wasn't the best timing for me. Linzi only had a few weeks left of her pregnancy with our second child and I was also concerned about having time off work when things were going well. Brad was also taking time off too, so I got cold feet, rang them up and pulled out of the tour.

I took to the new code and I would still be playing rugby

union now if things had been different. I really enjoyed it. I still follow Ionians and look out for their results every week. Union is completely different and not as physical for the backs – not as intense. At first I wondered what the pockets were for in the shorts. I was told that I would find out soon enough and, after playing the game, I realised there is a lot of standing around during the matches and in the winter you need to keep your hands warm!

11

Devastation

There was something wrong with me. I knew that. But in no way did I ever imagine how bad it was and how big a bombshell was about to be dropped on our lives. For months I had suffered with constant indigestion, a bloated feeling in my stomach and I had developed symptoms that made me see the doctor regularly without resolution.

My stomach had been getting tender and sensitive dating back to September 2005 and I really noticed how sore it could be when my son Taylor dived on me when we were playing together. Physically, I realised my fitness had deteriorated because at the end of my first year teaching at college I had beaten all the kids in the decathlon event. The following year we did it again, along with Brad Hepi, who was working on the course alongside me. There was a noticeable sign that all these kids had now gone above me and it was blindingly obvious that I had lost a lot of strength and fitness. I put it down to change of lifestyle, no longer training full-time and therefore, it didn't cause me any concern. However, it did not go unnoticed to others – people who had not seen me for a while started saying how much weight I had lost despite my reading on the scales remaining the same.

My physique was summed up when then Hull prop Garreth Carvell called me 'barrel chest and spaghetti legs'. Another day I was up at Hull Ionians where Hull FC were training and Andy Last took one look at me and told me I 'needed a good dinner down me'. It was not long after that I was diagnosed.

My stomach was becoming progressively bigger and because Linzi was pregnant with our second child at the time, we joked that I was coming out in sympathy with her but along with the other symptoms I was having we became increasingly concerned. I was still playing rugby union for Ionians and my form was noticeably affected by my condition. I felt guilty about telling the coach that I was not fit to play – that was shortly before I found out how ill I really was. The club really needed me and I felt bad because I couldn't give them what I previously had been. I felt like I was letting them down.

My GP was at a loss as to what was wrong with me, even after an endoscopy (a camera down my throat) during 2006. Although they could see some inflammation when they did a biopsy, there was nothing obvious and suggested it may have been a stomach ulcer, irritable bowel syndrome or my stomach producing too much acid.

They did not really know anything, so when I tested positive for helicobacter, a bacteria in the stomach, I was relieved because I thought they had got to bottom of the problem. I had two weeks on antibiotics, but when the problems returned the alarm bells really began ringing. Another doctor told me he was going to send me for a further endoscopy, but I demanded to see a specialist and asked if it would help if I paid to go private. Money talks and he said, 'Yes', that was on the Tuesday and I subsequently got an appointment on the Friday with a private consultant.

I went to hospital in the early hours of that Friday, September 8 with Linzi because she was having contraction pains. They put us in the delivery room but we only stayed there for 45 minutes before little Koby Zak Stephen Prescott was born at 1.42am. I tried to be there for Linzi, holding her hand.

I remember the birth vividly. The feeling when the little fella, Koby, came out made me well up with tears. It is probably because of all the worry beforehand, hoping that everything was going to be okay. After months of waiting and then finally seeing a baby born brings a massive relief so you have tears of joy. Linzi grabbed him straight away and said, 'Aw, look at him, he's beautiful.' And I felt exactly the same. I just could not believe it when he lay there on Linzi's chest.

We were a bit worried at first because Koby did not cry straight away like Taylor had done when he was born, but I put him on my chest and he was perfect. I arrived home at about 4am. Kim, the next door neighbour who had come in to sit with Taylor, jumped up straight away and I showed her some pictures that I had taken. I went in to give Taylor a kiss and he woke up so I told him that he had a brother. Taylor slept in my bed with me for the rest of the night. I was so happy that I had two healthy, beautiful boys and our family was complete.

When we woke up, Taylor and I went in to Hessle to buy some flowers. Taylor chose the biggest balloon for Linzi. We had to wait until visiting time to go back to the hospital which was late afternoon. Taylor was so excited to meet his baby brother but unfortunately, they only let the parents in outside of visiting hours. It was a long day waiting. When we arrived Linzi was up and about and, to my surprise, waiting to go home but the baby was asleep in the little cot.

I took some pictures of Taylor with Koby and we gave Linzi the flowers and balloon and everything was great. We waited for Linzi to get the 'okay' from the midwife and then we travelled home. When we got home everyone in the street came out wanting to see the baby. It was a fantastic feeling and none of them could believe Linzi was out so soon.

Paul, a neighbour from across the road, came over and we had champagne, fun and jokes. It was a great welcome home for the new addition to our family. The time ticked on and I had almost forgotten about my appointment to see the specialist at 6pm. I had to love and leave them and rush to the hospital so as not to be late.

I travelled to the old East Yorkshire BUPA hospital. I remember walking in thinking, 'What am I going to say about the money?' I had never been a private patient before, except during my playing days. That should have been the least of my worries.

Unfortunately, what should have been one of our happiest days as a family turned out to be the start of the most traumatic episode in my life. After five minutes I was called in to see Mr Wedgwood for the first time and he asked me for some history of what had gone on. He then he examined my stomach and abdomen. He did an internal examination and then I sat back down. Almost immediately, I knew something was badly wrong because his face had just changed. He told me straight that he was really concerned about me and wanted some emergency blood tests and CT scans done straight away.

He believed there was a possibility it was one of three things; lymphoma, internal hernia in the bowel or bad adhesions in the stomach but looking straight at me, said it was likely to be the first one.

This specialist said he could tell by my whole demeanour that there was something seriously wrong, even though he said it was unusual for someone at the age of 32 to develop the disease. It absolutely petrified me and I burst into tears as I walked back to the car. What was going on really hit me then and I realised I could have cancer but I still didn't know how serious it was.

All the time I was being given this awful prognosis, Linzi was back home laughing and joking, drinking champagne with the neighbours and a couple of friends to celebrate Koby's birth, completely oblivious to what was happening. The contrast could not have been starker – and our perfect world was about to be turned upside down and inside out. We could not have prepared ourselves for what was coming because when you are 'our age' you never think the worst.

When I phoned Linzi, I could hardly speak and just burst into tears before telling her that the consultant was really concerned. I needed time on my own and sat in the car crying. Linzi became upset too and said, 'Don't drive home, I'll come and get you.' I told her I would be okay and made my way home in a daze.

She met me at the door and gave me a big hug and then I went upstairs and lay on the bed feeling pretty numb and unable to take it all in at the time. Kim, our neighbour and close friend, took Taylor into the garden while Linzi began crying and asking me questions. She struggled to understand how the doctor could make these presumptions without really knowing me, when my own GP, who I had been going to see for over a year, failed to come to any conclusion. She decided to ring East Yorkshire Hospital to speak to Mr Wedgwood for clarity. He explained the situation. Linzi had initially thought it was simply a case of me looking on the dark side but the specialist merely confirmed the grim assessment.

It was so frustrating because despite seeing GPs for about a year, they had all missed it. I kept going over it in my head – how can a specialist see straight away that there was something drastically wrong and all those others see nothing? At the time Linzi and I comforted ourselves with the thought that the specialist may have simply been giving us the worst-case scenario. We thought, 'Let's not worry until we know what we are worrying about.'

This false optimism was further fuelled when my doctor, who I had been with for a while, came out to visit Linzi and the baby on the following Thursday and said, 'My money's on helicobacter and another course of antibiotics.' After my blood tests at Castle Hill, I had the CT on Thursday. I drank a litre of white chalky solution, which knocked me sick, and then they injected a dye into my body. This is something that I go through now on a three monthly basis and it has become part of my life. The nurse was quite chatty as I went through to the scan. After the first one she asked, 'Do you know that you have broken your collar bone?' and I explained and talked a little bit about rugby.

She took another two scans and then I knew there was something wrong because she stopped chatting with me. When I stood up the radiographer came in and started asking me questions about previous operations and asked when my follow up appointment was scheduled with Mr Wedgewood. They took the needle out and told me to go home. I could see in her face that something was wrong but I did not expect what was to come.

It usually takes about two weeks to get the results so when Mr Wedgwood's nurse practitioner, Rachel, rang the following day it was unexpected. They wanted us to go in to discuss my test results. Linzi answered the phone and she asked if it was bad news and the answer was a simple, 'Yes'. She then asked if it was 'really bad' and again the answer was affirmative.

They told us not to bring the baby because we would be going on to a ward but looking back I think it was because they did not know how we would react to the news we were about to receive.

Linzi told me it was bad news and got quite upset as she passed me the phone. I just thought to myself let's get there as quick as we can and hear the news. We knocked next door and again, Kim was willing to sit with the baby. On the way to the hospital we worked through the possibilities of what 'bad news' meant – whether that just may mean that I would need an operation. Perhaps we were whistling in the dark a little because deep down we knew it was not going to be good.

We walked across the car park holding hands and looked for

the ward '14'. We were buzzed in and straight away a nurse, wearing theatre blues, and Mr Wedgewood began to walk down the corridor to meet us. We knew it was a bad sign. I looked over to my right and saw a door labelled 'quiet room', and thought to myself, 'I hope I don't have to go in there.' Unfortunately, she said, 'Follow me' into that room and asked the nurse to bring tea in. All the time this was unfolding I was just thinking to myself, 'This doesn't sound good, this really doesn't sound good.'

It was a tiny L-shaped room and Linzi and I sat down holding each other's hands. Never in a million years were we prepared for what we were about to hear. Rachel, the nurse practitioner, was sat next to me when she delivered the results of the CT and blood test. In doing so she asked, 'Have you ever heard of metastatic cancer?' We shook our heads and then she elaborated, 'It means you have tumours everywhere in your abdomen and it is inoperable and incurable.' In explaining she used hand movement to underline the 'everywhere' bit. The upshot was that I had several tumours and I didn't know where to even start asking questions. Nevertheless, we asked away – it was more or less how long have I got? Can you not do anything about it? How come my doctors have missed it?

One of those questions was interpreted as, 'If you are asking me if you are going to see your boys grow up then the answer is no.' I can't describe the emotion I went through to think that I was going to die and not see my boys grow up. Those words ripped through me – it was like somebody had plunged a knife in my heart and ripped it out, and even now when I think about it I get quite emotional. We were both numbed by the words we were hearing and it was like it was not real – like we were watching an episode of *Holby City*. I would not wish anybody to have to go through that.

They left us alone for a few minutes whilst we came to terms with what we had just been told. I rang my mum and dad to tell them, and Linzi told her mum and dad too. Both Linzi's parents and mine had been over to Hull that week to see the baby but had gone back to St Helens. I told my dad, 'I'm not going to see my boys grow up,' and asked, 'What am I going to do?' He got upset as well and handed the phone to my mum. It was just awful. To hear my dad reduced to tears was also difficult because he was always so tough.

When the medical staff returned to the quiet room they explained that they could not find the primary tumour from the scan results, so I would need to have a Sigmoidoscopy, a minimally invasive examination of the large intestine, similar to a colonoscopy but not as invasive. I wanted this procedure carried out straight away, there and then, because I wanted to know immediately what I had. Perhaps even then I wanted to attack it, head on, get to the root of the problem so we could somehow move forward. They allowed Linzi to come in to the theatre because she did not want me to be alone – and she has been with me every step of the way since.

In the recovery room afterwards, I asked again for the best case scenario, looking for some hope to cling on to, The same nurse said, 'Months ... a year maximum. Don't worry you'll see Christmas.' Bearing in mind we were in mid-September, this wasn't the answer we were looking for.

All this sent me into turmoil. I was in shock, panicking and thinking about my two little boys and wondering how my family would cope. All the time I just kept thinking, 'Why me?' and I kept bursting into tears. They told us to go home and come back on Monday for further tests as the procedure I had just had was inconclusive. Linzi drove us home, but neither of us remembers the journey. I recall Linzi saying that we were going to have to be strong for the kids. I was in bits. Before we left the hospital car park I phoned my brother Neil, who immediately packed up and drove home from his holiday in Devon. Our whole family had been turned upside down.

What a weekend. The most shocking thing is we were given no support there and then at the hospital and offered no help from Friday until Monday. That weekend Linzi and I could have jumped off the Humber Bridge for all they knew about our mental state.

It was my eldest son Taylor's first full day at school and we were not there to pick him up. Linzi had to ring her good friend, Jemma Fletcher and break the devastating news and ask her if she would collect him. We felt guilty that we weren't there for him, something else to add to our worries. When we got home I went straight upstairs and lay on the bed but could not sleep, so went in to the spare bedroom and just cried and cried and cried. I was numb, devastated. I could not believe what I had been told and kept thinking that I was not somebody who was ready to die.

That night I decided I was going to have to go home to St Helens to face everybody because we needed help from family over there in order to be strong. When Taylor went to bed, I kissed him goodnight. I could not believe that I was not going to see him play rugby and football. I was going to be taken from my family and my thoughts turned to whether Linzi would be all right financially to look after two children on her own. I started adding up the finances and the shares and it made me re-evaluate. I must have only had five or ten minutes sleep that night because I kept waking up crying. I was physically exhausted.

At about 2am I went in and got Taylor out of his bed to be with me and I just hugged him and wanted to be near him. I stayed like that until the morning. All this time Linzi had to look after our new born baby. She was up doing night feeds, whilst having to deal with the weight of the world. She was helping to comfort me, stay strong and be 'normal' for Taylor and deal with the heart break that she was going to lose her husband all at the same time. The next morning came and I just could not get out of bed. Physically I had nothing left and I could not move. I managed to drag myself up but curled on the floor of the en suite. I didn't know whether I was strong enough to cope with this. Linzi got the kids sorted and packed the car up whilst I just about managed to get dressed and get in the passenger seat. We drove home to St Helens. Another journey we don't know how we managed to get through, but one we needed to make to keep Taylor occupied and try our best to protect him from this nightmare.

All the way home I was silent, drained and unable to speak. We had the radio on and Taylor was spotting well known lorries, the same thing he did on all the return journeys over the M62, only this time Linzi and I didn't join in. We met Linzi's mum and dad, June and Peter, at the Black Bull car park on Knowsley Road and they took Taylor to the circus, which was taking place at the Saints' ground. All this was an effort to shield him from what was going on because he was only five years old. I could not look Linzi's parents in the eye because I thought I had failed them by not being able to look after their daughter and their grandsons. That is how I felt at the time.

From there we went to my mum and dad's house. As I walked in my dad burst into tears. Neighbours Mary and Les were there and I went through and sat down with my head in my hands. Everyone in the house was devastated. I went upstairs and just cried. Neil, my brother, came round and told me I had to fight it, but all I was thinking at the time was I had no hope, no life and I had nothing in my body to fight. They had put me in a dark tunnel with no sign of a light at the end of it.

My close friends Mike Ford and Paul Barrow came round to see me and they could not believe it. Paul brought a copy of Lance Armstrong's book round. They were trying to make me positive and give me some motivation but from what I had been told I had nothing. For all that I hoped, prayed and wished I needed a start line. When Linzi's parents came round they came up and told me I had to think about fighting it for my boys. I apologised to them but told them too that I needed a light to be switched on. They were very supportive and reassuring. The whole of that weekend my good friends came to my mum's to see me. They all rallied round and were there to give me support. Old team-mates phoned as the news started to spread around the town. It was good to know I had such good friends and family.

We travelled back to Hull on the Sunday, with my mum and dad following on the Monday to support the children whilst we attended more appointments and procedures. We had been told, until biopsy and investigation, to believe what the specialist had told us. You don't think it is bullshit or a best guess, so we believed I only had a few months to live. On returning to Hull, I was back in bed still finding it very difficult to come to terms with the surreal situation. Linzi had the difficult job of ringing other close friends to break the news before they heard it from somebody else. I was unable to face the world. As soon as Linzi rang to tell Steve Crooks, my old coach and friend he said, 'I'm on my way!' Crooksy came up to my room and more or less made me come down and sit downstairs. He was great and said to me, 'Steve, if you have got one day, one week or one month I know you will fight it.' That is what helped motivate me and was just what I needed to hear. I was a wreck but he came in and kind of picked me up. When he was talking to me he also mentioned cyclist Lance Armstrong and all the other people who had fought diseases before. I just broke down in front of him, which I had never done before. He was great and both Linzi and I feel that this was a real turning point in the way I was going to handle this.

He coaxed me to leave my room, go downstairs and sit with Linzi and our new baby. It wasn't the best start in life for Koby. He had been brought into the world at a really difficult time but he was still loved very much and helped me to put some fight into this battle. The realisation dawned on me that I had to fight if I wanted to see Koby smile, walk and talk. Meanwhile word had got out about my condition and somebody from the *Hull Daily Mail* tried to speak to me at my house to ask me how I was feeling. Reporters have a job to do and the paper was great with me while I was playing and since my illness – but there is a time and a place. I called Steve Crooks and he had a word with them to give me a bit of space and they did.

My mum and dad arrived mid morning as we had to be back at the hospital for a colonoscopy. This time they put me to sleep. In the recovery room, the doctor came to tell us that although they had found the colon to be clear they had found some inflammation on my appendix from which they had taken a biopsy. I told the doctor that I had my appendix removed when I was 12 years old due to an abscess. He went on to say that he was aware of this, however, for some reason a small stump remained at the end of the colon and it was this that showed some slight abnormality.

Before I was allowed to leave the hospital, nurse practitioner Rachel explained that I was going to have to have a biopsy taken from the abdomen the following day. She advised that I would be admitted for a few days whilst they did this and carried out further tests. She showed us the films from the scan and pointed out the tumours within my abdomen. She went on to tell us that, in fact, there may be some form of treatment available to me but they would know more after the planned tests. She also told us that the scan report had also come back. We were shocked to hear that they hadn't got the report before they delivered the devastating news the previous Friday. They only had the scan pictures and probably shouldn't have told us what they did as it was only their best guess. I think they panicked when they saw how widespread the tumours were throughout my abdominal area.

On leaving the hospital I felt a little more positive. The fact that treatment was now a possibility gave me a boost. It was only a small thing but it was something for me to cling on to – it gave me some hope. On the Tuesday I went for a biopsy on the same ward where I was first told the bad news. They put me in room 9, ward 14 – a dirty room, with blood on the floor. 'That blood is not mine,' I complained, so they asked me to leave the room while they cleaned it out. Although I told the trainee taking my blood that I was frightened of needles he then cocked it up, taking five minutes to put a cannula in. It was a day of waiting around in one room after another. While I was waiting for the biopsy in the Ultrasound Department, the same one we had been in only weeks earlier for a growth scan on our unborn baby, there was an old woman screaming in the background, 'Why don't you let me die? It is too painful. I don't want to wake up.' I desperately wanted my life, but she didn't want to live. To hear that was a strange feeling to say the least.

After my biopsy we asked for counselling, and attended a session on the Thursday before I got the results. At that session they told us nothing is concrete until we get the results and told us to try and be positive. I only went a couple of times, but after that they let us get on with it. We also found out that there was an oncology-counselling department, which is what we really could have done with on the day we were first told the bad news. Nobody had told us it was there and apparently we had to ask for it.

On Friday September 22, Rachel rang to tell me that there was some light at the end of the tunnel and asked if she could come round to our house. She explained that I had pseudomyxoma peritonei, telling us it was very rare and that nobody at Castle Hill Hospital had any experience of it. She had gone on to the internet and researched, printing some mortality rates off and again, ever the optimist, told us I had three to five years to live rather than months as I had previous been told. It all depended on whether it was low grade or high grade because my biopsy had not yet determined this. So, although I had received more positive news there was still a dark prognosis, but we were elated that there was more hope.

Rachel explained that there were two specialist centres for this rare disease – Washington DC and The Christie in Manchester – and she said she would arrange a referral.

12

It's a Waiting Game

We were told nothing about pseudomyxoma peritonei so basically Linzi and I said to ourselves, 'Let's get cracking and find out about it.' We went on to the internet and printed off all the information and facts. I had to wait five weeks to see specialist at The Christie. It is such a rare disease, with only 150 cases a year that they only review once a month and I, typically, had just missed a review. In the meantime, Castle Hill was still our main point of call and I continued to see them on a regular basis.

The more we learnt about the disease on the internet, the more questions we had. We took these questions back to Castle Hill as we could not wait, what seemed like an eternity, to ask the people who would have more answers. Rachel tried to explain to us by showing us a scan of a 'normal abdomen' and then showing my scan. She explained that all the black dots I could see on mine showed the widespread disease. It helped me understand a little bit more what I was dealing with.

I learnt that pseudomyxoma is a slow progressive disease – so I kept wondering how long I must have had it. There were signs I suppose, maybe like at Hull Sharks I was not getting any abs even though I was training hard all week. Or when I had a groin operation in 1996 when they said I had multiple adhesions and my intestines were stuck to my stomach wall. There were perhaps signs that could have been identified earlier. It was said on a few occasions that perhaps I had had it for 10 years plus.

Again we knew nothing concrete at this stage and were left to our own devices again. I made a few calls, Steve McNamara came round regularly and helped organise a meeting with a surgeon from Leeds who knew about pseudomyxoma peritonei. Geoff Lane, who is originally from St Helens, came over from Leeds and met up with us at the Village Hotel in Hull to talk us through what I was looking at.

It was just nice to speak to someone who knew about what I was suffering from. As soon as he met me he recognised the features – the thin face, skinny arms and fat stomach and said that there was no doubt I had pseudomyxoma. He explained what he knew and told us of a specialist in Basingstoke who had a great reputation. He asked if I would like him to arrange an appointment with him, but at that stage we were two weeks into waiting for The Christie. If we went south for treatment it would be a case of leaving the children up here.

It was so refreshing to speak to Geoff and he restored a little bit of faith in the medical profession and could tell us in layman's terms what was happening to me rather than the apparent guessing game that had preceded it. Geoff was so helpful and the meeting was very beneficial for us.

As time passed I was deteriorating. Linzi was so worried that she rang The Christie and spoke to the pseudomyxoma manager. She explained her concerns and told her how hard it was being in the unknown. She asked if my scans could be looked at before the meeting. Mia was very helpful and understanding. She told us that the surgeons were in theatre but she would ask them if they would have a look at them. True to her word, she called back the following day. She reassured Linzi that the scans had been read and that there was 'nothing surprising' on them. She explained how slow growing the disease was and advised that my condition would not be getting any worse in the time we were waiting.

Speaking to Mia helped give some reassurance and hope to Linzi because she was going through it too. 'Nothing surprising' – that was surely a good thing to hear from somebody who knows what they are dealing with. It helped us both get through the next weeks because we felt if they were not alarmed, like the specialists in Hull, then there must be something they can do.

So after a long wait, we finally went to our appointment at The Christie. All I was looking for was some hope to cling on to. We were in the waiting room for what seemed like an eternity. Both Linzi and I were so nervous, stomach in knots and unknowingly tapping our feet, anxiously waiting to see the consultant. All through the wait, different professionals had told us what a good surgeon Miss O'Dwyer was. We had heard nothing but positive things about her, so we were confident she was going to give us the hope we so desperately needed.

We were called through from the waiting area and asked to wait in yet another room. Every time a door opened I would feel sick thinking they were coming to me. Finally, a young consultant, Mr Paul Fulford came into the room and introduced himself. That was our first disappointment. No disrespect to Mr Fulford and nothing against him, but we had heard so much about Miss O'Dwyer that we really wanted to be under her. The consultant was very nice and he explained about the disease and about the major operation which they offered as a possible cure. He went on to tell us that this wasn't an option for me as the disease was so widespread.

My head was a mess when I asked him what actually was available to me. He offered to do an operation to clean things up which would make me more comfortable. We had done our research leading up to the appointment and knew what I wanted – the 10 to 13 hour operation which would get rid of the alien that was growing inside of me. So I asked him how long the operation he suggested would take. 'Two hours or so,' he replied. There were so many thoughts going through my mind – but two hours? What could they get rid of in that short time? I know it is stupid to judge on time, but that was all I could think about. Linzi could tell from my questions that I wasn't satisfied. It was a massive disappointment to us both. Linzi started asking questions and trying to push for more. Was there anything else that could be done?

I asked if there was any hope, and he suggested there was a chemotherapy trial. That gave us a little bit of light but to be honest once he had told us that I could not have the big operation to remove all the tumours, I switched off. All we wanted was the big, cure all, operation.

Then they told us it would be another three weeks before they could do the operation. Linzi broke down, and told them we could not wait longer because we had already waited five weeks. They could see how desperate we were and then said they would do it on the following Tuesday. It was hard all round. We then had to go home and tell the family that I could not have the big operation we had prayed for. We were all back to square one.

Linzi was determined though and would not accept what they had told us. She rang Washington DC and spoke to the secretary of Dr Sugarbaker, who had pioneered the operation. His secretary told us to go to Basingstoke, gave us the name of the surgeon and could not speak highly enough about the PMP team there. She told us that if anybody could help us it was them. They had learnt all they know from Dr Sugarbaker. We remembered what Geoff Lane had told us, it was the same surgeon's name that had come up again, Brendan Moran and his team.

Linzi immediately sourced the number and rang them. She managed to get through to the team and amazingly the specialist nurse told her that the surgeon, Mr Tom Cecil, was around and that he would speak to her. He listened to the story so far and said, 'I'll see you tomorrow at the end of my clinic.' We were so grateful. We picked my scans up from The Christie, which was quite awkward. Going for a second opinion surprised them, although they did manage to prepare the scans for us to pick up on the way down to Basingstoke that same evening.

When we got to Basingstoke the first thing they did was thank us for coming to see them. It made me just wish we had gone to Basingstoke when Geoff Lane recommended it and although the five weeks would not have made a difference health wise, mentally it would have done.

Mr Tom Cecil showed me the scans and talked me through them and agreed with The Christie in that they did not think they could get all the tumours, but said they won't know for sure until they got in there. However, they offered do a lot more debulking than The Christie had. It was when he said they would give it their best shot that some hope was restored. He proposed to carry out a five to six hour operation that would still leave me with a good quality of life. He explained that they could take away everything, which would really affect my quality of life and still not cure me, which would not be advisable. They told me go away and think about it, because it would mean three weeks in hospital and time away from my very young family.

Suddenly, I had a big decision to make because The Christie had squeezed us in on the Tuesday and it was hard to tell them that we were not going. I wanted them to get rid of as much as they could and Mr Cecil at Basingstoke gave us a date in three weeks time.

To be honest the team at The Christie were not too happy, but Linzi explained to them why we had chosen this route. There was then a bit of confusion when The Christie told us that if we went to Basingstoke that we could not go back there for chemotherapy. They explained most people settled for one or the other – either the big operation and then sit and wait or a small operation followed by a chemotherapy programme. We wanted to put the two together, they resisted at first, which frightened us because I would need chemo in future and thought I may be cutting my ties with them.

I suppose we wanted the best of both worlds, and Linzi could not get her head around why they could not give us that and pleaded, 'This is somebody's life you are dealing with.' Eventually, The Christie were persuaded and said, 'Okay then, go to Basingstoke and we will discuss treatment options as and when.'

It seemed to us that they didn't get many patients asking for a second opinion and it worried us that they may hold a grudge in the future but we had to do what we thought was the best for me. Even after we had made our decision to go to Basingstoke, we still had disappointments. The pseudomyxoma nurse rang to say that Mr Moran, who we had heard so much about and who had been recommended to us, because of his reputation, was going to be at a conference in Australia. We thought, 'Here we go again' and once again Linzi got upset on the phone, saying we really wanted Brendan Moran to be there. However, we were reassured that Mr Cecil had learned everything off him and was an excellent surgeon. We were happy with that. I just wanted the best chance possible and to be honest we really liked Tom Cecil when we met him. Then they suggested bringing my operation forward so Mr Moran could be there too. They did everything for us. The new date for the operation was now November 14, 2006.

Despite all that, Geoff Lane still told us to ring Washington to see if they could do the big operation to just get it clear in our minds that we had left no stone unturned. My hospital in Hull sent my scans and we followed them on the tracker. However, Dr Sugarbaker's clinic asked for a $250,000 deposit but said they could only give it their best shot too, which was no different to what was being offered at Basingstoke. We could have got the money together by selling the house, but we would have ended up with nothing. I had the boys to think about.

Fair play to the Americans, they were really good and regularly gave their advice to Linzi for free. Likewise Geoff Lane, who was doing this off his own bat, not as part of his job. I explored every avenue and used every contact I had to get the best possible treatment. The advice I give to people now is never settle for a bad diagnosis, go away and do some research because it is your precious life and you have to do what you can to preserve it.

There was a lot of preparation needed before I had my op. It wasn't like it was being done locally. We had to sort things out for the children. It was agreed that Linzi's mum and dad, June and Peter, would look after the boys. Linzi's sister, Sarah, did lots of ringing round to try to organise schooling for Taylor whilst he was over in St Helens. We didn't know how long we would be there, but we couldn't allow him to miss school for three weeks while we were in Basingstoke. St Julie's Primary agreed to accept Taylor as a guest pupil at the school. It was local to Linzi's parents' house and the same primary school she had attended as a child. That was one less thing for us to worry about. They agreed he could stay there for as long as we needed. With that in mind, we thought it would be wise to plan to stay over that side of the Pennines after the operation, close to family, while I recuperated.

Koby was only nine weeks old when I had my operation, so we had to take everything but the kitchen sink over with us. We decided we would stay with family until after Christmas. With the operation being brought forward a week, it meant we didn't have time to settle Taylor into his new school as we planned. It was literally a quick hour visit with Linzi on the Friday, before he started on the following Monday, when we would have already been in Basingstoke.

We knew people, old friends, who had children in the class he would be going in. We had been in touch with them and they asked their children to look after Taylor and make him welcome. On the visit, it was reassuring that they all gathered round him and all wanted to be his friend. This really helped not only Taylor, but Linzi too. She felt really guilty for not being able to take him on his first day and also guilty for leaving both the boys for such a long period. We had never left them before. This added to the stress and pressure of an already difficult situation but we knew it had to be done.

Leaving the children was heart-wrenching. Koby was so young, Linzi was worried that he wouldn't remember us when came back. Taylor was only five years old, but he was obviously more aware of what was going on. How would he cope without us? How would he cope with his new school? It was Sunday, November 12 when we had to leave for Basingstoke. Both Linzi and I fought back the tears when saying our goodbyes to the boys. Linzi drove us down and I was admitted that same evening.

Mr Moran and Mr Cecil came to talk to me. I was very nervous about the operation and was trying to convince them, 'Look, I'm fit. I can cope with it. Get rid of as much as you can.' Both surgeons said it depended on the op and what they found, but they assured us that it would be their best shot. If they thought they could get the lot, they would do it, but not if they were not sure, because they wanted me to maintain some quality of life.

We had done our research so we asked if I could be given the heated chemotherapy whilst on the operating table. We knew this was usually only given if you had the full operation, but I wanted the opportunity to destroy as much of this disease inside of me as possible. They gave me no guarantees but said again they wouldn't know until they knew exactly what they were dealing with. I was surprised to be told that there was another guy with pseudomyxoma in hospital waiting to have the operation on the same day as me. The disease is so rare, I just didn't expect that. They went on to tell me that they thought they would be able to perform the full operation on him as they had caught him early enough. They explained that I would be meeting him the following day whilst they showed us around intensive care areas. They did this to try to prepare us for what to expect when we came round from theatre. It also helped Linzi as it gave her an insight as to how I would look, with lots of tubes and machines attached and how I would be cared for. They also explained that the two surgeons were going to be operating on both patients at same time. I was amazed, but by doing it together they would get different opinions. Tom Cecil would be my main surgeon with Brendan Moran popping in and assisting.

I knew it was going to be a big operation and they had informed me that one in five may die on the operating table. So before leaving for Basingstoke I sat down on my own and wrote letters that could be opened if anything went wrong. They were really deep letters to be honest, and I thought it had to be done to say goodbye to Linzi and my two sons. It was horrendous doing that and even just writing about it now makes me quite emotional. That just shows how nervous and frightened I actually was.

13

Hope

They came to take me down at 7.30am.

I had a medal of Our Lady attached to a piece of cloth, which had been given to me by a very close friend's mum. It had been passed on to lots of people who had been ill and they had all felt it had helped. I am not that kind of person to be honest, but in these circumstances I was thankful for anything that gave me hope. I clung on to it all the way down to theatre, squeezing it with one hand and holding Linzi's hand tightly with the other.

They allowed Linzi to stay with me in theatre until I had fallen asleep. This is something we had never heard of before, but we were both grateful for it. They did everything to try to help us get through this emotional, unthinkable ordeal.

The anaesthetists told us that they would ring Linzi during the operation to let her know how it was going. Linzi, my mum and my dad all sat in the hotel, staring at the phone on the table, waiting for the call. When they rang at 1pm, they explained that they could not do the big operation, but told Linzi they had done some extensive debulking and I was stable throughout. They advised that they should start to make their way back to the hospital as I would be out of theatre shortly.

Mr Cecil and Mr Moran spoke to Linzi and my parents before they were allowed in to intensive care to see me. They told them that they were pleased with what they had done, taking 10 kilos of tumour out of my body. I had coped well and they explained to Linzi that this would give me an extended and better quality of life.

They were all upset because that faint hope of the big operation to cure me had gone but I had asked them to give it their best shot and they did.

The surgeons went on to explain to Linzi that I had been through a massive operation and they were going to try to keep me asleep over night. However, minutes after that the surgeons reappeared, laughing, saying I was already awake. I think they all knew what my character was like by this point, I wasn't going to back down, I was going to fight it all the way. All I wanted was a pen and piece of paper to write down my many questions. I could not speak because there was a tube down my throat and up my nose, which was making me heave when I swallowed. The first question I wrote down was, 'How long was the operation?' This was so I could try to determine how much they had removed and if they had managed to do the 'big one'. I also put down a big thank you to Linzi and told her how much I loved everybody. It was very emotional but I was so relieved it was over and I had come through.

The surgical team came round to see me when I had come round fully. They explained the operation and informed me that they had removed 80 per cent of the tumours from my abdomen, pelvic area and the lining over my liver. They took away my spleen, so that does not help me fight infections anymore, and removed my colon and some of the small bowel and partly cut away some of my stomach. Due to the extent of the debulking and the removal of the large intestine I was left with an ileostomy. I found this very difficult to come to terms with. My body was never going to be the same again. In response to my many questions the surgeons told me that the work was done to put me in a better place, get rid of as much as they could and help me to live as long as possible. They had to make the decision, while I was in theatre, to leave me with a permanent stoma. I don't think I have ever got used to the fact, however I have learned to live with it and manage it in the best way I can.

On a positive note, the surgeons told me that I had been given the heated chemotherapy whilst open on the operating table. They had taken onboard my plea and it was something that the Americans had told me to fight for. I was thankful that I had been given that.

Even though I lay completely flat, tubes coming from everywhere, hooked up to all kinds of machines and covered in bruises from where I had been strapped to the operating table, Linzi and my mum both thought I looked more comfortable immediately after the operation than I did leading up to it. I guess a lot of the apprehension and stress had gone now, as well as 80 per cent of the disease, which was taking over my body.

They initially told me that I would be in intensive care for five days but I was out after 24 hours and put into a side room on the ward. Although Linzi was concerned, the medical staff saw how I was recovering and realised that I did not need somebody sitting at the end of my bed 1:1 giving round the clock care. I am glad I was in an individual room; I am a private person who likes my own space. My head was not in the right place for general chit chat with other patients. I needed to put all my energy into getting myself right.

Because I was in my own room, Linzi decided to stay at the hospital. She was worried about leaving me in case I needed anything so she stayed in the chair next to my bed. I was given all sorts of pain relief, an epidural and a PCA where I could control how much relief I needed. I was given Fentanyl in the PCA and told to keep pressing the button for the pain even if I didn't really need it so that it didn't build up. The healthcare assistant advised Linzi that it had been known for some patients to have a reaction to the drug and one of the side effects was to hallucinate. Well it's a good job that Linzi had the tip off because during that night I was horrendous. I believed that I was on a merry-go-round and I was trying to get off, but I had just had a major operation and had staples from my breast bone to my pelvic bone and was supposed to be lying flat. Linzi was frightened by my behaviour as it got progressively worse. I think at first she was laughing at me and taking mental notes so she could have a go at me when I was back to normal. She was reassuring me all the time, telling me it was normal due to the medication, however, in her own mind she was frightened. In the end she had to buzz for assistance. We did laugh about it once I was swapped onto morphine instead, but that was a feeling I never wanted to have again.

My recovery continued to progress at a good speed. So much so, Linzi arranged for her mum and dad to bring the boys down for a visit. This was a massive boost for me and helped with my rehabilitation. The physio had been round trying to get me up and about, but I didn't really have much motivation. I knew I had to be able to walk a mile around the wards before I would be allowed home. So when the boys came, I would go for a walk with Taylor, who was five at the time. We would use the time to talk about what he had been doing at school and with his grandparents whilst I had been in hospital.

It was great to see the boys. We had told Taylor that I was not very well, that I had a sore tummy, early on. We had tried to prepare him for what was about to happen in a way that would protect him. He was so resilient. He was a good boy and just got on with whatever was thrown at him without any fuss. Our new son Koby was a perfect baby, as good as gold and did not cry for the first six weeks of his life. He never made a murmur, almost as if he knew he had to be good to help us. He continued to be good whilst he was being cared for by his grandparents and whilst in Basingstoke. We were so proud of them and thankful to them that they didn't add to our worries and stress at that time.

When the physio returned, she was surprised how far I had come. I went for a walk and ended up climbing all the flights of stairs, to the top of the hospital above and beyond what she had wanted me to do. There was no stopping me and after that she didn't need to see me again. She was happy with my progress and my fitness.

From then on, I just wanted to get home, I was up and about. People could not believe how well I was coping. I shocked my family and friends with my progress and I left hospital on Tuesday, November 26, one week ahead of schedule.

I was still very weak and my body was still a mess on my discharge, but I was happy to be going home. I left hospital with so many tablets and instructions. I had to take antibiotics daily, for the rest of my life, because my spleen had been removed in the operation. This would help my immune system and help to protect me from illness as much as possible. That was just one of many tablets, which now have become a daily routine for me.

Before we left the hospital I was given the results from the histology. It revealed that I had low grade pseudomyxoma, which is the best news I could have had in the circumstances, even though I would never be free from the disease. I had made it through!

14

My Family, My World

My wife Linzi has been an absolute rock for me – all the way through the highs and lows of my playing career and especially during my illness. We met when we were very young. We both attended the same school, De la Salle and even though it was located on two different sites – boys on one and girls on the other – I still managed to cross the brook for certain lessons.

Linzi had liked me for a while but she never made it known. We used to go to the same parties and one night I walked her home. We were only about 14 or 15 at the time. From then on we started seeing more of each other and we went out quite a lot in a mixed group, my friends and Linzi's friends. We used to go to discos and to the cinema quite a bit. In the beginning it was the usual teenage boyfriend and girlfriend on/off relationship but it quite quickly developed into something more. I used to go round to her mum and dad's house every night. My dad would drop me off and pick me up until I was old enough to drive and then I was always asking my parents if I could borrow the car.

We had a good social life and lots of mutual friends so we all stuck together. When I started playing in the 'A' team and more importantly, the first team, our social life suffered as we couldn't go out drinking. That's probably when we became more serious. We were still only teenagers but we spent a lot of time together. The only thing we could do on a weekend was to go to the cinema, so Showcase Cinema on the East Lancs Road became our weekly jaunt.

We were soon inseparable and planned our first holiday abroad together. Linzi had just started university and I was just breaking into the first team at Saints. We saved up and spent a fortnight in the Dominican Republic. We had a ball, all inclusive, nice hotel, we got on great. We vowed to continue to work hard and enjoy good holidays as much as we could, something that we have continued to do to this day.

In 1996, after the Wembley win, I decided it was time for me to buy my first house and move out of my family home. I was 23 years old, I had saved up some money and along with my winning bonus from the Challenge Cup Final it meant I had enough for a deposit. Linzi played a key part in helping me find my first home. We knew that one day we would be sharing it together, but at the time Linzi was still studying at university so we wanted to get the timing right. From the day I got the keys, Linzi stayed most nights but we didn't make the full commitment of moving all her belongings in. I suppose we still wanted some independence. We were still young and we didn't want to rush things.

On August 30, 1997, I proposed to Linzi – it was nothing romantic because that's not my thing – I simply asked the question out of the blue. Linzi was very shocked and began to cry with happiness – I hope. She did say, 'Yes' and we went ring shopping but we probably had the longest engagement ever due to my rugby commitments. By this time, it was summer rugby league and we did not really have time to plan a wedding and we were still both young. Our relationship continued to grow though and Linzi supported me all the way through my career. She watched all my games, both home and away and put up with a lot of crap. It's not easy living with a professional sportsman, especially if things are not going well. If we lost or if I didn't have a good game then I would get pretty moody. I was always very critical of myself and as a consequence, was very down on myself if I had made mistakes. Linzi had to deal with that, try and talk me round and put up with my sulks. You see the glamorous side of players' wives and girlfriends, not so much in rugby but sometimes people do liken them to footballers' wives. It's not like that at all. People don't see the difficult things, like having to put up with their other half being away on pre-season tours, international trips, injuries and job insecurities.

When I left Saints to move to Hull, Linzi left her job with IBM in

Sale to move with me and managed to get a transfer onto a customer site at Immingham Docks over the Humber Bridge working as a computer analyst. It was sort of a promotion for her, which was good, but it was something else she had to adapt to.

We moved to Hull in the winter of 1998 and we were only given two weeks to find accommodation. However, Linzi was still working full-time in Manchester which meant we only had two weekends to find a place to live. I knew it was important to find somewhere decent for Linzi to be happy. We were used to having a nice home and I knew she wouldn't be able to live just anywhere.

Most estate agents were closed weekends, so the first visit to Hull was us driving round looking for 'To Let' boards and peering through windows, and that was only when we were happy with what we had seen from the outside. I clearly remember thinking she is not going to go for any of these. 'Look at that carpet,' she would say.

'We'll get a rug' I would respond, trying to make light of it. In the end we had to settle for a house that was too big for the two of us just because the carpet was clean and it was in a nice area. It was a four bedroom detached newish house, just on the outskirts of the city in Brough. We still had to get my dad to paint it and decorate it using his skills from his days with the council. Linzi and her mum spent a day cleaning it from top to bottom before we moved.

This was the first time that we officially moved in together. Although Linzi had been staying at my house for a while, she hadn't officially 'moved out' of her parents' house. It was the start of our new life together. We had to start again – our friends were left behind in St Helens, we both had new jobs. It was different for me because I got embedded in a team with a strong social side involving lots of drinking and going out. Linzi had to make friends through the wives at the club, as the job she was in was very male orientated and she worked in an office full of blokes. It was a big step for us but you make the best of life and get on with it.

We loved our time at Hull Sharks. We became very close as we were on our own over there, we only had each other and we became best friends. After two years, when the club got into financial trouble, I had to move clubs again. We decided that we would stay in Hull and I would commute rather than starting all over again. We were happy and we had made some very good friends. I am so glad that we made that decision as we had to suffer similar problems again at Wakefield, less than a year later. All the insecurities could have caused a strain on our relationship but they didn't, if anything all that upheaval and uncertainty probably brought us even closer together as a couple.

At the end of 2000, I luckily secured my return to Hull FC. 2001 was going to be a good year for me. I was content with my life, happy to be back at Hull, I had played in the World Cup, rugby was going well and I felt ready for the next chapter in my life. After returning from the Ireland camp (I had been away from home for a few weeks), Linzi and I felt that we were ready to start a family. We were both aware that the wedding still had to be arranged and it was something that both of us wanted to do, but we didn't want a winter wedding and it wasn't the most important thing to us. We were living like a married couple and we were happy as we were. We decided that we would try for a baby, if nothing happened after a few months, we would put it on hold and book the wedding. We went on holiday to Jamaica. As soon as we came back Linzi knew she was pregnant. She took the test and it was confirmed just before Christmas. We were both elated. We decided that we wouldn't tell anybody until we were sure everything was okay. We went back home to St Helens for Christmas and it was so hard not to share our news with all our family. Once Christmas was over it was easy as we didn't see them all again until after we had had the scan. Our families were delighted. This would be the first grandchild on both sides.

Both Linzi and I were keen to find out what we were having, not because we had a particular preference, but because we are nosey and also wanted to start buying things. We didn't think it was fair to spoil the surprise for everybody else so we told everybody that we hadn't found out the sex. That was how we left it until the baby was born.

Taylor Cameron Prescott was born on September 7, 2001 in Hull Maternity Hospital. At the birth your emotions take over, you see the pain that the women go through. Linzi was brilliant and handled it really well. She was very calm and didn't shout or have a go at me like I had been warned. Everything changes when a child is born, especially when it's the first one. When Taylor came in to the world I burst into tears. To think I had created a life, it was so special. He was amazing. We were so happy to have our little boy, our son. What a feeling!

I picked Linzi and Taylor up from the hospital on the morning of our last game of the season. I dropped them off at home and had to go to the game. After the match, I went out with all the lads, wetting my baby's head. Linzi had lots of visitors, both sets of parents had come over and also her friends came round to meet the new addition to our family. She was happy for me to go out but I'm not sure she was too happy that I brought my team-mate, our friend Logan Campbell, back at 3am to meet the little one. She didn't say anything but when I sobered up I thought maybe it wasn't the best idea.

There were lots of babies born at the club around that time. Logan Campbell, Richard Fletcher, Gareth Raynor and Jason Smith all had babies within a few weeks of us. Match days were like a crèche but it was good socially as we were all in the same position. Taylor was very active, even before he was born he used to kick the life out of Linzi. We used to go out with all the other families and they couldn't believe how hard Taylor tried to get up on his feet, he couldn't keep still. He was only weeks old at this point, but he still has lots of energy now. He was a very quick developer. He was walking at 10 months and seemed to be ahead of his time in everything he did. He is a very athletic child; we could see that from a very early age. He would always have a ball in his hand, whether it be rugby or football. He always wanted to play, and to be honest I was lucky enough to have the time to spend with him. I used to always be passing and catching with him. I would take him in the garden when I came home from training and kick the ball around. He was, and still is, sport mad.

When he was four years old I took him to a local sports centre where they did futsal sessions (Brazilian football). He loved it and really concentrated. Most of the other kids his age were just playing about, putting their tops over their heads or putting the balls up their jumpers, but Taylor did what the coach was telling them. I also used to take him to the Village Hotel swimming. I taught him myself. He would swim the length of the pool in no time. He obviously had the sporting gene and could turn his hand to anything at such an early age.

Linzi struggled going back to work after having Taylor. We had no family around and so he had to go to nursery. Linzi used to cry when she left him and felt really guilty. Taylor did settle after a while but he started to pick up lots of illnesses. It was complicated, Linzi couldn't keep taking time off work and I had to be at training. When he got chicken pox at 15 months old and we were trying to juggle everything, we decided it was time for her to become a full-time mum. We realised that we were lucky enough to be in a position to do this and Linzi made the most of it. She made sure she spent quality time with Taylor, teaching him to read, to write his name and numbers. It was the best thing we did. We felt we gave him the best possible start to life.

It wasn't long after Linzi finished work that I suffered my career ending injury playing for Lancashire. It was a difficult time for us. We not only had financial worries but we also had the worry about what I was going to do after rugby. I was at rehab most of the time trying to get myself fit again, so I guess life at home wasn't much different to when I was training, but Taylor really missed watching me play. On his second birthday he was mascot for Hull FC. It was sad for me that I wasn't part of the team on that day and Jason Smith, the club captain, carried him on to the field whilst I was watching from the tunnel.

Once I had finished rugby and started working at the college I began to think about getting married. We had no obstacles in the way now and it was something I wanted to do. We were over in St Helens, having a family meal for my dad's birthday, my parents, brother and sister-in-law and my sister were all there. I had been thinking about it for a while. I went to the local florists and bought some red roses and put them in the boot of the car. When everybody was seated for the meal, I nipped out and sneaked them in. Nobody had any idea what I was about to do. I mentioned earlier that I am not a romantic person, so I shocked everybody, especially Linzi, when I pulled out the roses and asked her to set a date for the wedding. Linzi cried again! It was probably more of a shock than the first time I had asked her, but I'm so glad I did.

After lots of searching on the internet, looking through wedding magazines and countless journeys across the Pennines to the North West, looking for the right venue, we found the perfect place for us. As soon as we drove up the sweeping driveway of Shrigley Hall in Cheshire, we knew it was where we wanted to have our special day. We were worried that we would have to wait a long time for an available date, but we were delighted when the wedding co-ordinator advised us of a cancellation 14 months later, on Saturday August 6, 2005. I left most of the organising to Linzi, although I did get involved in all the important stuff and I've got to say that we wouldn't have changed a thing on the day. Everything went to plan and we had all our family and friends there. It was perfect. Taylor, almost four, was the star of the day. He thoroughly enjoyed himself and announced to everybody during the wedding speeches, that he was glad his mum was now a Prescott, which brought tears to most people's eyes. I had two best men, my brother and my best friend, Mike Ford. They did a joint speech and really embarrassed me but that's all part and parcel of the big day. I wouldn't have expected anything less as they were only paying me back from when I did them the honours a few years earlier. Linzi looked beautiful and I was very proud to call her my wife. She was a great mum to Taylor and I knew that we were going to be very happy. After all, we hadn't rushed into anything; we had been together for 15 years and engaged for eight of those.

We jetted off on honeymoon the following day. The three of us spent the next 12 days in Mauritius and then four days in Dubai. We had an amazing time and absolutely fell in love with Dubai. It has since become our favourite holiday destination and we have been back several times. Our boys love it.

When we got back home, back to reality, it didn't take Linzi too long before she started thinking about another baby. We were married now and she thought that the next natural step would be to complete our family. I was happy as we were, just the three of us, although I knew I always wanted another baby I was hesitant at this moment in time mainly due to financial pressures. However, Taylor would be starting school in 12 months time and Linzi didn't want to go back to work and then have to finish again if we did decide to have another one. Having a baby was hard work; we were just getting our life back. Taylor had always fitted in with our life, our routine, from the minute he arrived. He had to. We had no babysitters in Hull so everywhere we went, he came. Would it be that easy with two? I didn't know if I wanted to go back to the sleepless nights, not that that was really my domain. I knew if Linzi returned to work and got back into her career it wouldn't be fair to ask her to give it all up again. We talked about it for a little while and decided that there probably is never going to be a good time, there would always be a hurdle. We didn't want Taylor to be an only child so we decided to give it a go. It was probably a case of now or never.

Again, we were very lucky; it didn't take us long before Linzi was pregnant. She did the test on New Year's Eve. We didn't tell anybody again, so Linzi had to pretend to be drinking when we went to our friend's house to celebrate the New Year. Linzi's sister Sarah had just announced that she was expecting her first baby, so we didn't want to take the shine off that. The due dates were only two weeks apart.

This pregnancy wasn't as straightforward as when she was carrying Taylor. Linzi was very sick and lost a lot of weight. We waited until after the first scan and then told Taylor, who in turn shared the news with our families. He was delighted that he was going to be a big brother and revelled in the chance to tell everybody.

Again, we decided to find out what we were having, we didn't mind as long as everything was okay and the baby was healthy. Most people say it's nice to have one of each, but I think if we were honest, we both wanted another boy and that's what the scan confirmed. We were thrilled, a little brother for Taylor.

Koby Zak Stephen Prescott was born on September 8, 2006 at Hull Women and Children's Hospital five years and a day since Taylor had come into the world. I now had two beautiful boys with Yorkshire roots. We were overjoyed. Koby's labour was much quicker than Taylor's, in fact we had only been at the hospital for 45 minutes before he was born. It was still very emotional and we were over the moon with the new addition to our family. Taylor was delighted with his brother.

Koby didn't have the best start in life, as the timing coincided with my diagnosis, but I can honestly say that I don't think he has suffered as a consequence and it certainly hasn't affected him. He has always been given so much love and I probably have shown more affection to the boys because of my situation than I would have done otherwise. I make sure I tell the boys and Linzi that I love them every day. It is important to me for them to know that.

Koby hasn't known any different. I am his dad, he never knew me, or should I say remembered me, without my body defects. On the other hand, Taylor was old enough to see the changes I went through, he just accepted them. It's funny though as it is Koby that has the most questions. I am glad he feels comfortable asking me and I try to answer him as honestly as I can. I want to be open with them about my differences; it is good for them to see that not everybody is the same and that my body is different. Hopefully, it will help them to respect others and not prejudge people.

Both of the boys' lives were disrupted by my diagnosis, but we tried to keep it to a minimum. The move over to St Helens was probably the biggest change, although it was also for the best. They were now near to their grandparents, who had missed out on so much of their lives, especially Taylor's.

Being back in St Helens meant the granddads could get involved with Taylor's sport. He was five years old when we moved and we started taking him to football on a Saturday morning at Bleak Hill Rovers and rugby at Thatto Heath and he loved both. Although he was only still young, I used to play a lot of Playstation FIFA football with him so he knew how to tackle and would be flying in, slide tackling. It really brought him on and I could see he had something special. He also enjoyed his rugby. He had obviously been brought up with rugby from a very early age and he had a keen interest in playing the game.

He played for a year at Bleak Hill but he could not play matches because he was only five, so I moved him to St Helens Town. During his first session there, a scout, Steve Leather noticed his talent and asked if we would let him go to the training camp for Blackburn Rovers, which was at Sutton High on a Wednesday evening. There you get six weeks to show what you can do – and then Liverpool came to watch him and we were asked to take him to their satellite group at Kirkby.

The big football clubs are scouting the kids at a very young age – we also went to Man City, Bolton, Burnley and Everton with Taylor. It was all 'show me some skill'. It was very difficult at Liverpool – from a six week trial you go into a shadow group and if you are good enough you get picked up. He was in the shadow squad for ages.

He ended up getting in the main 7/8 age group squad at Liverpool – it was all about getting a contract then. We thought we would keep our options open – and took him to Everton and in the first game he played he scored seven goals. They really liked him. This was just before they gave the contracts out – the Reds and Blues were both interested. It was a hard decision for an eight year old to make.

During this time, Taylor had to make a decision. He had been playing both rugby and football and had a sporting commitment most nights of the week. I told him he had to make a choice. Carry on at Thatto Heath and choose one football team or concentrate totally on his football, where there seemed to be more options. It was hard for him, but we were worried about the physical effect it would have on his body if he carried on the way he was going.

He was lucky enough to be offered a contract at both Everton and Liverpool. This was a choice that only he could make. Taylor made his own decision to go with Liverpool. That was the team he supported and loved, so we understood his decision. He signed his contract in April 2009. He is still with them and we are so proud of what he has achieved.

I am pretty critical as a dad – possibly too much so, maybe it's because I want my boy to be perfect. Sometimes I have to step back and think, 'He's a child not a robot' and there are ups and downs. I wanted him to be perfect as a player, but he is only 11 years old and kids can't be perfect all the time. I sometimes don't realise how good he is.

He is very committed and still loves his sport. He trains four times a week and then plays a game. He sacrifices a lot for football and he shows amazing dedication and has already played in Europe against the likes of Juventus, Ajax and Bayern Munich. Having coaching at a top class level is quite something for a lad of his age – his kit is better than the kit I got when I was a professional. I was gobsmacked when he came home with two lots of Predator boots, double training gear, wet jackets, tracksuits and polo shirts– it was more gear than I ever received as a pro and he is only a kid. We do keep him grounded because he perhaps in some ways does not know how lucky he is to be getting the training that other kids don't get.

Academically, he is very bright too – he must get that from his mum – but Linzi did a lot with him when he was younger.

My youngest son Koby is also very bright and doing very well so far in school. He is a character and makes us laugh. He is different to Taylor though, he isn't as obsessed with sport. I suppose he is just a normal seven-year-old. He has just started playing rugby at Thatto Heath and he is enjoying it. It's great to see him following in both mine and Taylor's footsteps. It is here where we have seen his desire to win. Although he has competed and won in school sports days, this was just fun. At rugby, he is only playing with the cubs, u6s, but every week he is desperate to win the trophy which is given to the star player so he plays his heart out. Lately, he has also started becoming more interested in football, playing with his friends and cousins, but he isn't quite ready to play for a team yet. Watching him, he looks like he may have a natural talent and sport probably is in his blood but it is whether he wants to apply it. His love is watching films but that may change as he gets older.

I will be happy with whatever my boys do as long as they do their best and they are happy. They make me so proud every day. It is very hard when I'm playing with my kids and I think, 'What would I do without them?' and 'What would they do without me?' It is very emotional. We try to protect them as much as we can to give them a normal life. They don't ask too many questions about my illness; all that we have told them so far is that I have a poorly tummy.

We knew we were in for a difficult time with the kids. We had to be really careful with how we managed things; we switched the telly off or talked loudly over it, if ever they were talking about me. We knew there was going to be a time when Taylor needed to know more. One of his friends said to him, 'Your dad is really poorly isn't he?' He told us that, but we said, 'You know that I've got a sore stomach, don't you?' We told them that I'm going in for scans but I suppose they didn't really know what that means. As Taylor is getting older, he is becoming more aware and has started to show his emotions a bit more. I have frequently been admitted to A & E with bowel obstructions, and he has been fine with it, but over the last few months he has started to get upset when he sees me going in. He can probably see the pain I'm in and now understands more. Koby is less bothered and gives a cheer when we tell them I have to go in, not because he wants me to be ill but because he loves staying at grandma and granddad's house. He knows no different really because it is all he has ever known and I would much rather he react in that way than worry about me.

He knows I always bounce back and Taylor is also fine and copes remarkably well after the initial upset.

I'm sure it must be awful for him to see me in such pain but we always reassure him and both the boys have been very resilient which makes us very proud of them.

At times I would say to Linzi, 'Do I tell them or not?' because it will be a massive shock to them when finally something does happen to me. It is very difficult and upsetting – I won't lie, I do think about the time when the worst does happen and I am not here for them anymore. We started reading information provided by Macmillan and contemplated getting counselling to try to prepare us and guide us through doing the unthinkable. It's something that has to be done, but something Linzi and I are dreading.

Dealing with my illness has made me appreciate my wife a lot more. Linzi has been through so much with this and I would not have been able to fight it without her support and strength. When I was first diagnosed with cancer it must have devastated her more than me but Linzi is a good girl and I would not be here, where I am now, without her.

I was only 32 when I was diagnosed – the prime of my life and at a time where you don't think things like this are going to happen to you. When I was utterly devastated and left bewildered by the news, Linzi was a big help in taking the burden, and even now she probably doesn't realise how much she has been through herself.

Linzi has continued to support me on all my challenges even though she sometimes wishes I didn't put myself through so much. When I think up new ideas for challenges she always says, 'This one is unachievable, why make them harder and harder?' She knows what I'm like though and lets me get on with it. I always prove her wrong!

What we have been through makes me appreciate my wife and realise how much I love her. I hope that Linzi and the boys are proud of my achievements. I feel like I have shown them how hard I have fought to be part of their lives and share their experiences. I hope they are as proud of me as I am of them.

My family is my world.

15

My Journey

After the operation my main aim was to recuperate the best I could. I knew I still had disease within my body and that was hard to come to terms with, I desperately hoped for a cure but I was determined to get myself back to some level of fitness, although at the time I didn't know what that level would be or how I would progress. Firstly, I had to build myself up and put back on some of the weight I had lost. I had dropped from 12 stone 7 to 9 stone 7 which was quite drastic. I know people, especially women, think it is easy to put on weight, but when you have to it's not that straightforward. My weight loss and subsequent new frame shocked most people when they saw me, and some didn't even recognise me. When I felt stronger, the first thing I did was to buy a completely new wardrobe. My waist had gone from 34' to 30' and my clothes were hanging off me which made me look even more poorly.

There were many changes to come to terms with when I got home and it wasn't only my weight that had changed. My body was now different and I had to adapt to that. The major thing for me was the stoma. For example, I had always slept on my front pre operation, but I could not do this anymore. For weeks I could not sleep because I couldn't find a position which suited me and the changes to my body. My eating habits also had to change because of the ileostomy. I could no longer eat high fibre foods and had to cut out any nuts, seeds, certain vegetables, sweet corn, mushrooms, fruit skins and many more things to help keep me out of trouble. I was given guidelines but I had to find out slowly what was right for me. As a rule of thumb, basically all the things I loved were now off the menu. I was very self conscious of the stoma and made a decision that I would try to keep it private. Most of my family and close friends were aware but I never discussed it with them and I made it clear from the start that I didn't want people to know. It wasn't because I was ashamed of it because after all it was a medical necessity for me and was helping to prolong my life, but I was embarrassed about how people would react. I thought people may see me as a different person. I had to get used to it myself, it was still new to me. I also think this was one of the reasons which made it so hard for me to put weight on as food would pass through so quickly.

At Christmas time the scales did start to move in the right direction and I could see a physical improvement. By January I was feeling marginally stronger and it was time for me to go back to Basingstoke for my follow up appointment. Tom Cecil was pleased with my progress and he had already made contact with The Christie with regards to treatment and possible chemotherapy. He advised me that they like to leave it for six months post op to ensure I was back to full strength. The Basingstoke team were happy to refer me to The Christie Oncology department from then on.

It was time now to consider moving back to Hull after spending my recovery period with family in St Helens. It was a frightening thought. We had had so much support, especially with the children, from Linzi's parents which allowed her to spend more time caring for me and helping me to recover. From then on we would be on our own.

When we moved back to Hull it was nice to be just a family of four again, allowing us to spend quality time together. Taylor returned to his original primary school, St Andrews in Kirkella.

Although things returned to normal pretty quickly – I continued to progress, both with my weight and my fitness – Linzi and myself discussed possibilities for the future. We knew that further treatment was imminent and that it would be over in Manchester. After a lot of thought we decided it was going to be a logistical nightmare travelling back and forth across the Pennines and juggling childcare with appointments. We decided that we would make the permanent move back to St Helens. The boys were missing their grandparents and we would need some help and support, after all we didn't know how I would react to the chemo. It made sense, however we loved living in Hull and had some great friends there. It wasn't an easy choice to make.

We put our house on the market and planned to move into the house we had already bought with the intention of renting it out in St Helens. Although things were improving on a daily basis and I was getting on with my life trying to be positive and trying to accept what I was still going through, I still had bad days. Well to be honest it was the night times which were the hardest to deal with. When it is quiet and you are lying in bed going over in your mind what has happened and worrying about the future. It is not easy. Linzi helped me tremendously and still does. She knows what I am thinking just by the sighs that I unknowingly make. Although it's not quite the same for her, she is still living it too and probably has the same thoughts and fears. She listens to me and tries to make me see the positives. I'm sure there are times when she doesn't know what to say to help me, but she always finds words of reassurance and that really motivates me to get my mind back on track. It doesn't really take too much, perhaps going back to being a sportsman, I had to pick myself up after so many knock backs and I'm sure that has helped me.

It wasn't only words of encouragement from Linzi but I also received so many cards and letters of support from people wishing me well. Joe Walsh, a local businessman and friend, sent me a diary and he wrote in it: 'To Ste, a private place to store your thoughts and keep fighting all the way to victory. Hope this helps. Let me know when you are ready for book two'. This is the diary that I used when I started penning this book. Ian Connor, a former team-mate from my early days at Saints, wrote me a long letter to try to pick me up. There were lots more, too, and I still have all those letters that people were kind enough to take time to write to me. Each and every one of them meant so much to me and my family. I found comfort in reading them and they gave me the motivation to continue my fight.

The sale of the house was quicker than we imagined and things moved fast. The appointment for The Christie tied in with the move and things fell into place.

By April I was back to 12 stone and I had met with the consultant,

Dr Mark Saunders. He was brilliant from the start. He arranged for me to have a scan as a baseline and he gave us some advice. He told us to get it into my head that I could not be cured. Once we had come to terms with that it would be easier. He gave us stories of hope. He gave us positive scenarios of his patients with PMP and arranged for us to return mid month to commence treatment.

I was nervous about going on chemotherapy. Who wouldn't be? I was aware of all of the different side effects but I didn't know how I would respond as everybody is affected differently. All I was sure about was that it would attack both the good and the bad cells within my body which was pretty scary. With the chemo I was going to have – Mitomycin C combined with Capcetabine – I was told that my hands and feet would become sore and blistered and my mouth may be affected. These, along with tiring easily, were the effects it had on me. I have to say I tolerated it well overall. Beforehand I had read Lance Armstrong's autobiography in which he describes his chemo and the side effects he experienced, like coughing up tar. The mere thought of that was horrendous, so I considered myself very lucky. Lance's chemo was a much more aggressive form to the one I had but when you hear the word chemo you class it all the same but there are so many different ones with so many different side effects.

I'm not saying it was easy for me; again I had to look at my diet and eliminate even more foods. You have to be quite regimented when you are having treatment, particularly with your eating habits, timings of food and also what you can and cannot eat. For example takeaways, soft cheeses, shellfish. In fact when you are having treatment you can say you follow the guidelines of a pregnant woman to some extent. For me it was a restriction of more foods that I love, but hey that was a small price to pay if it was going to help control or even reduce the remaining disease.

The treatment consisted of an infusion over 30 minutes once every three weeks in the Chemo suite at The Christie and then large tablets twice a day for two weeks. After a week off the tablets to give my body a rest, the cycle began again. I did this for three months. I was then scanned to see what was happening inside and if the treatment was effective. The scan revealed the disease was still stable and they could actually see a slight reduction in the size of the tumour over the liver. I was delighted with the results;

any reduction was a bonus even if it was only small. I had another three months of the same treatment but half way through my feet began to get really sore. Dr Saunders decided that he would reduce the dosage for the remaining cycles. I wanted to continue at full strength because I thought it wouldn't be as effective, but you have to listen to the experts. He explained that the side effects were a sign that it was too toxic for me so it had to be reduced as it would not have been good for my body. It was reduced by 20 per cent and I did tolerate it better. At the end of the 12 cycles I was scanned again. Stable disease was the result and Dr Saunders had no way of telling whether it was the treatment or my body fighting the disease. It was decided that I would have a break from treatment and see what was happening in another three months and how the remaining disease was behaving.

The three monthly scan results kept coming back as stable disease. The best I could have possibly wished for. I knew I was never going to be rid of this alien within my body so keeping it at bay was a positive for me. As time went by the scans stretched to four months apart and eventually to every six months. This was a great sign but it also scared me as six months is a long time and a lot could have happened – but it never did. The results kept coming back as stable. This didn't stop me from worrying though, especially as scan day and results day approached. I feel nervous each time and get a sickly feeling. Sometimes I actually suffer from abdominal pain in the days leading up to the results. It's funny what the mind can actually do because as soon as I get positive news those pains quickly disappear.

All the time I am looking for hope. Every time I hear on the news about a medical breakthrough for certain cancers, I stop and listen to see if it could benefit me. Family members cut articles out of newspapers and magazines and pass them on to me to read. In the early days every time I had an appointment with Dr Saunders I would ask him about gene therapy, injecting straight in to the tumour, or anything else I had heard about in the media. Pseudomyxoma doesn't behave like most cancers so he would explain why these therapies were not suitable for me. I realised that Dr Saunders was very knowledgeable and if anything new did come out he would tell us but it doesn't stop me having hope and searching for a miracle.

As the time passed by I slowly began to get my head around things. I think we live in a little bubble. I can't say you ever forget what you're going through but things became easier to deal with. The fitter I became and the more challenges I completed the better I felt. I believe that having the focus of the charity and believing that my body can achieve has definitely helped me fight this illness. I have often used the phrase 'you don't know how strong you are until being strong is your only choice'. I believe in this.

I guess I have become a little complacent over time and because I have been doing well, I kind of expect my results to be good too. I do still get nervous but not as much as Linzi does. I suppose it's my body and I know how I feel. Linzi is always so relieved to hear positive results and, don't get me wrong, so am I, but I probably would be more shocked if they were any different. The disease is under control, it will always be there but I will never give up fighting. Having said all that, I still experience side effects from the disease. I suffer from small bowel obstructions on occasions. I think quite often people read about me in the paper or see me in the gym or completing crazy challenges and think that I am fine, not many people witness the pain and other suffering I go through.

In 2009 I suffered my first bowel obstruction and didn't know what was happening. It frightened me and I was rolling around on the bathroom floor in agony. The out of hours doctor quickly diagnosed the problem and sent me to A & E. My local hospital, at this point, didn't know me or anything about this extremely rare disease.

Prior to this setback I had been great but I had relaxed on the dos and don'ts on what foods I could tolerate with the ileostomy. I had slowly begun to introduce things into my diet and I think having a kiwi fruit was one step too far. The hospital x-rayed me to see if I had a mechanical obstruction and gave me fluids to prevent dehydration. With some morphine to help with the pain I had to sit it out and the obstruction cleared within a couple of days.

When Dr Saunders found out about the obstruction his instinct was to get me back on chemo. He explained to us that the remaining disease was around the small bowel and it must be this causing the bowel to narrow and thus causing the obstruction.

This chemo was slightly different to the previous course. It was infused over a longer two-to-three hour period on ward 5 of The Christie. Along with the infusion, oxaliplatin, once every three weeks I also had the large capcetabine tablets for two out of the three weeks like last time. Having to go back on treatment was a big blow, because I was back to feeling great again after the obstruction but if it was going to help I had to do it. It was another six months of poison in my body. During the treatment I suffered from effects of the cold and it being a snowy November didn't help things. I had to wrap up more than normal even in the house and I even bought hand warmers to put in my gloves and wore woolly hats when I went out. It also felt like I was swallowing glass when I drank anything colder than room temperature. I was probably more tired than during the first lot of treatment I had but other than that I tolerated it okay.

When I have a bowel obstruction, whether it is complete or partial, I suffer from acute abdominal pain and my stoma stops functioning. I can now tell myself as soon as the pain kicks in and my abdomen becomes distended that I have a SBO and I go to A & E mainly so they can control the pain. Every time I endure an obstruction it sets me back a little and knocks my confidence. You could say that the little bubble that we live in is burst for a short period. It is sort of a wake-up call reminding us that I still have PMP. We know now what is happening and that I will be okay in a few days which does make it easier for Linzi and me to deal with, but as our boys are getting older they are starting to ask more questions and realise what is happening.

Another aspect of the illness, which people won't realise, is that the tumour produces a mucin. This jelly like substance builds up inside of my abdomen and collates in pockets. This is a very unpleasant consequence of the disease that I have had to learn to deal with. Periodically, these pockets make their way to the surface and a hole appears in the skin and the mucin, clear jelly, is forced out. When this happens I worry about infection from having an open wound, but I manage them well. I have to be very careful as having no spleen leaves me wide open to infection because I don't have a good immune system. It was quite a shock when the mucin first came out, but my theory is 'it's better out than in' so I try to squeeze as much of the bad stuff out as I can.

Although I do have these hiccups along the way, they are few and far between and generally I live a normal, active life. I have probably got myself to a level of fitness that I haven't achieved before. Obviously, being a professional rugby player I was fit but through the challenges I have completed since founding the charity I have trained my body to accomplish a new level. This just shows that anybody can train the body to do something and it will respond. It is a matter of preparation and commitment – that is key to anything in life. The fact that the disease remained stable for such a long period of time could have been because I was keeping myself mentally and physically in shape and focused.

16

A Little Help from My Friends

The Rugby League community has always responded brilliantly when called upon to help various causes, as I have since found with my own Foundation. Yet, I was staggered to find out after my initial diagnosis, that people would be organising fund-raising activities for me and my family. I think I was waiting for my operation at the time and Richard Swain, a good family friend, came round to see me and he mentioned that Lee Radford was in contact with Stuart Fielden and that they wanted to do a boxing match. Although I really appreciated the proposal, I had a lot on my plate at the time and didn't really want people to feel sorry for me and feel like they had to do things for me. I wasn't being unappreciative of their offer; I just didn't want to trouble anybody.

Lee Radford had heard about charity boxing events in Australia, involving Tawera Nikau and Mal Meninga and he thought of doing something similar over here. He phoned Stuart and the fight was on, to take place on February 2, 2007.

Mike Smith, a friend of Steve McNamara, was the organiser and he did an amazing job. He organised absolutely everything and took time off from work to make sure it was done properly. He had not done anything like it before. Things gathered momentum from there. The clubs and their coaches, Peter Sharp and Brian Noble, had given permission for the two players to take part, which was absolutely brilliant and it was just a case of finding the venue and taking it from there. The event was switched from a suite at the KC Stadium to the Hull Ice Arena, with a capacity of 2,000.

Mike didn't involve me too much in the organisation of it all because I was recovering from my operation. Both Lee and Stuart took the whole thing really seriously and looked in great condition on the night itself. Radders had been trained by Mark Elwood, the kick boxer from Hull, who organised the rest of the bill for us, which were kick boxing bouts. He also put himself in the ring too and came out of retirement to fight for the British title belt.

So Stuart and Lee did come to blows during what was called the Rumble by the Humber. The contest lasted until 30 seconds into the second round when Lee caught Stuart with some cracking shots early on and his legs finally gave in. I said to Stuart afterwards that the defeat didn't matter and I wanted just to thank him for what he had done. It must have been tough for him facing the wrath of the 'home' crowd in Hull – a bit like Ricky Hatton going over to fight an American in Las Vegas. This showed what kind of character he is to put his reputation on the line and get in the ring for me. Lee was very emotional after the fight had finished. Typical of him, he had put everything into it and it certainly wasn't about the winning, I'm sure the result wasn't the most important thing to him.

Although I was still really poorly and weak, it was a fantastic night and very well-supported by the likes of Brian Noble, Steve Ganson, Barrie McDermott, Terry O'Connor, Nick Barmby and loads of former players from Hull and Wigan, who made up part of the huge crowd. I couldn't thank everyone enough for what they did on behalf of me and my family. It was certainly a ground-breaking idea and proved to be the inspiration and springboard for other events we have organised on behalf of the Foundation.

When I was first diagnosed with cancer I had a lot to come to terms with, mentally and physically. I soon became aware that I was not alone and people were trying to do things to help me. At that time I had been given only months to live and so people, who I did not know then, began staging fundraising events to give my family some financial security and take that one burden away from me. Initially, they organised some forums at local social clubs in the St Helens area.

Martin Blondel, who was a regular Saints fan, had watched me play but had never met me, was the driving force behind this fund raising. He spoke to Mike Denning, now the chairman of the Steve Prescott Foundation, and began to take things further. After the forums and when I was out of hospital, they decided to hold a gala dinner at the Hilton Hotel in St Helens. It was an opportunity for me and Linzi to meet the people who had done so much for us. It was probably the first time I had been out in public since my operation and I was so nervous that I almost changed my mind but we didn't want to let anybody down. Meeting Martin for first time that evening made it a special evening for me – what a rock he has turned out to be for me and the Foundation. He is like family to me now. I did not know Martin before my illness, but he has been absolutely superb and has taken over our lives in some ways. To do so much for somebody he did not know makes him a true Saint.

Other people also excelled on that evening, donating things for the auction. Former Saints winger Chris Smith gave up his 1999 Grand Final ring which went for £800. Prior to that Tommy Martyn had donated his 1996 Challenge Cup medal which was auctioned on ebay and sold for £2,700 to Paul Stanton, who had seen the story in the *Liverpool Echo*. After he won the medal he contacted Martin and said he wanted Tommy to have it back. It was decided between all parties that the medal would be donated to the Rugby League Museum. What absolute magnificent gestures – and they were not alone. When you receive the sort of devastating news I was given, it changes people – and it certainly changed me. You change your ways and look at life differently.

It didn't end there. Martin came up with the idea of a Legends game. It was not going to be any old game; Martin wanted to get Saints' 1996 Wembley winning team together in which I had played full back – and they managed it apart from Simon Booth and obviously Keiron Cunningham, who was still playing at the time. Chris Joynt had been Martin's first point of contact to see if he could get the players to agree. They all turned out voluntarily and made it a very successful day.

Our team of Wembley winners took on an All Stars team which included some big names but I had no part in planning it – it was all down to Martin, Mike Denning and Dave Howarth. Opening up a ground like Knowsley Road is a costly affair and the organisers had to make an early decision – restrict it to one side of the ground at a cost of £800, which would have held 1,500 spectators or open up the whole ground at an expense of £4,000. With two weeks to go until game day, some 400 tickets had been purchased in advance. The committee could not decide what option to go with so they asked for my input. All that I could say was, 'I don't want anybody turned away on the day'. The decision was made; Knowsley Road would be open to full capacity. The match sold out all of the corporate places and Elite Homes sponsored the jerseys. The attendance was the most pleasing aspect with 5,793 filling four sides of the ground.

I was not in the best of physical condition at that time and I had just started chemotherapy. Martin told me that all I could do was to kick off the game and then I would have to leave the playing area. No way! My argument was that all these lads had turned up to play – and fans had turned out in big numbers – frail as I was, the least I could do was stay on the field and give it my best. I did the first 20 minutes. Even then I didn't want to come off – Dave Lyon, the bloke I replaced in the Saints first team all those years ago was on the touchline beckoning 'come off'. He didn't want me to overdo things, but also I know he would have been desperate to get out on that pitch himself.

One of the highlights of the day was seeing my eldest son Taylor, who was only five at the time, turn out and score for the All Stars. It was a planned move where he had to run the ball back and finish with one of my trademark dives. However, before that Gary Connolly had urged Vila Matautia – one of the Saints' biggest hitters in his day – to tackle Taylor on his way through. So when Taylor came running through, Vila pushed him and he went flying to the ground. The crowd was in uproar, but fair play to my boy – he still managed to keep hold of the ball, got up and ran the length of the field, rounding the full back, me, before completing a flying dive under the post.

As for the game itself, it was all set up to be a two handed game of touch beforehand because there were a few players struggling with injuries, but then Bobbie Goulding intervened. Bobbie, who has always liked the physical aspect of rugby league, went in to the opposing dressing room and declared, 'We are playing tackle!' And boy did Bobbie make the most of that licence and he put a massive shot on Gary Connolly. It was a perfect opportunity for Bob to settle a few scores. It was a good event and I was really pleased that so many people had made the effort. Former London player Tulsen Tollett, who I had roomed with on the Great Britain tour to New Zealand in 1996, even flew over from Ireland to take part. The fact that these lads had turned up and were willing to play meant a lot to me.

At first I didn't want to make a big deal of anything – but when I saw the work they had put into it, it made me realise I had to stand up and do as much as I could. I just remember looking around and being moved with the variety of club shirts in the crowd – fans from Leeds, Wakefield, Hull and Wigan rubbing shoulders with Saints supporters – it was overwhelming. That day played a massive part in the challenges I went on to do later. People had done so much for me it dawned on me I was not finished yet and I could do something to inspire other people. While I was still here I wanted to do what I could. Yes, I was frail. I had lost a lot of weight having been through a major operation and having organs removed but it gives you such a lift when you realise people are willing to help you and you see thousands backing you. The rugby league community certainly showed me that day that they were going to be with me every step of the way for my battle against cancer.

They gave me ideas, too, and after recognising how successful the Lee Radford-Stuart Fielden bout had been, the Steve Prescott Foundation went on to organise its own boxing events.

That started in June 2008 when we enlisted former rugby league players to fight at the Reebok Stadium, Bolton. We realised we could not do it with present day Super League players so we thought about a different approach and turned to those who had hung up their boots. Getting players to don the gloves was an altogether tougher assignment. We were probably priced out of the market for Martin Offiah and even offered him £10k to box Alan Hunte because of their history of wing rivalry going back to their Wigan-Saints days. We chased Chariots for a bit until he replied, 'I am a dancer not a fighter.' He was doing *Strictly Come Dancing* at the time.

To be honest he was not the only one that was wary about getting into the ring – after all we were only a little charity, particularly back then, but there was also a fear about getting injured and how much of a show they were going to make of themselves in a boxing ring. They had nothing to compare it to. However, some former team-mates and opponents were more than willing to undertake 10 strenuous weeks of training to take part in the contest under the tutelage of the World Celebrity Boxing. As part of the training, the contestants even visited Ricky Hatton's gym in Manchester, when Ricky himself gave his full support for the event. During this period of training all the boxers were assessed and matched up to the same standard opponent to create competitive fights on the night. The fights themselves were well policed by former World Champion Steve Collins, who was instructed to stop it at any sign of someone getting hurt.

Among the bouts were Steve Hampson and Anthony Sullivan, former Super League referee Karl Kirkpatrick and Jason Donohue. My brother Neil, who trained in kick boxing, wanted to take part and he fought Chris Smith. Smiggy said he was just going to go for it – throwing haymakers and bombs, you name it. Although Neil jabbed Smiggy throughout – and left him with a bloody nose and lips – he had been knocked down during the second round when the ref called break; as a result the ref judged it Smiggy's way. Neil was absolutely fuming not to get the decision after being so technically superior over the contest.

Maea David 'fought' Esene Faimalo, but the lads had been brought up together and didn't want to hurt each other. Brad Hepi lost to Oldham chairman Bill Quinn, who had boxed as an amateur and Alan Hunte, Garry Schofield, Warren Jowitt and Tim Street also took part.

On the night itself I entered the ring and took on former British and European middleweight champion Herol 'Bomber' Graham in an exhibition bout which delighted the audience. Robbie Paul had been the scheduled opponent for the exhibition bout but he had to be withdrawn due to playing commitments, I had no hesitation in gloving up. I had been on holiday for a fortnight and when I returned I only had time for one session of four two minute rounds and I did a bit of work on my stance.

Despite his age, Herol was on form that night, and Andrew 'Wolfie' Pahlen, a friend and Hull FC fan, took him on first. Wolfie trained really hard leading up to the night. He had raised a lot of money for the charity and didn't let any of his sponsors down. He took a good account of himself in the first round. I took over from him and had a go in the second round and we both jumped in and took him on in the third and final round. It was all a bit of fun.

Initially, I had it in my head that I wanted to go in and land some punches – that was a challenge because Herol was notoriously hard to hit, and was famed for his powers of evasion. However, just before he went to the ring, he came over to me and said, 'Listen, I have got a detached retina so don't hit me in the face.' Where else was I going to hit him? It threw me a little! All these people had turned out so I thought I'm going for it anyway. So I managed to get him in a corner and attempted an uppercut, I narrowly missed – the entire crowd were shocked. Then I feinted with one and hooked with the other and managed to land one, against the odds. He quickly called me a bastard and then jabbed me back straight in the abdomen. That wasn't in the script.

It was a great event which, despite some teething problems, raised £32,000 together with further awareness and publicity for the Foundation as it got some good coverage. After the success of that several National League clubs, such as Featherstone, Batley, Hunslet and Dewsbury provided players and we staged another boxing event at Batley Frontier in April 2009, and it raised £16,000 for the Foundation. Once again local communities were brought together for such a worthy cause.

Due to the success of the previous events, we decided to put on another boxing show in St Helens. After searching for the right venue, it was decided that we would transform Sutton High Leisure Centre into a glitzy boxing arena. A lot of hard work went into organising the night, we had to hire caterers, organise a bar, put up lighting and install a dance floor. We finished off the look with black star cloth and candle-lit tables to make the audience feel like they were in a high class auditorium.

Steve Collins, who had refereed the previous events, was double booked so John Conteh stepped in. Scouser John, who was a former World light heavyweight champion in the mid seventies, let the fighters get stuck into each other. It made for a brutal boxing night and everyone was surprised; it made it an exciting evening. However, it was only for charity and my heart was in my mouth at times especially when Bernard Dwyer and Tim Street threw bombs at each other throughout the three rounds. The main bout was two natural born winners. Brian McDermott, former Marines champion, the class act and Paul Sculthorpe, the boxing enthusiast, who had been sparring for six months. Two very different approaches to boxing produced a clash that had the crowd wishing there were 12 rounds rather than three. Brian's better ring craft proved the key. The party piece was Herol 'Bomber' Graham taking on Warrington's Richie Myler and Paul Wood, individually then together. They managed to land punches on the slippery Sheffield fighter but he never winced. We raised £20,000 for the Foundation.

17

Walking Against Cancer

The idea behind doing the first Trans-Pennine walk came about because everyone had assisted me and so I wanted to help other people whilst I was still physically able to. It was Martin Blondel's brainchild and it came out when we were attending a charity match between Saints and Wigan supporters at Robin Park. We tossed a few ideas around and then Martin eventually came up with the idea of the walk from Hull to Old Trafford taking in all the Super League clubs along the way.

Although we asked the doctors' opinions before setting off, as long as I was feeling physically fit and able I was going to walk regardless of their advice. The doctors at The Christie said they were fine with it anyhow, because they had seen how quickly I had recovered from my operation. I was in good shape for it and they could see that for themselves.

My job was simply to get myself mentally and physically right, the planning was down to Martin. I don't know how he managed to pull off the organisation involved because it was all new to him, yet he did an amazing job. Martin sorted out the route, sponsorship forms, media, people, advertising, transport and support vehicles as well as contacting the police forces in all the towns where we were walking.

As the big first day in Hull approached I became a little nervous about whether I was in good enough shape and particularly about the numbers who would turn up. The *Hull Daily Mail* came to see me on the eve of the walk and wrote a feature that allowed me to pour my heart out, talk about my illness and explain how I was feeling. This was the first time I had spoken openly about what I had been through. It was emotionally draining but I was glad I had done it when I read the article the following day and I hoped me doing this would help other people.

The first day from Hull FC to Ionians was a very difficult stretch because I had to meet all the walkers for the first time and deal with the media. The pleasing thing was seeing people wearing both Hull and Hull KR jerseys, with supporters putting aside their rivalries for two good causes. I was joined by ex-Saints team-mate Anthony Sullivan, fittingly a Hull lad, Shaun Briscoe and Richard Fletcher. The latter two went on to complete the whole walk with me. As we moved through the streets of Hull, people came out to chat and were putting £20 notes in the buckets. It was a shock to me how generous people were and as we walked from west to east Hull there was no difference in people's responses.

Although I wanted to talk to everybody, it slowed me down and I was unable to take a break. It took its toll towards the end and I was quite tired, my quad and calf muscles were sore and some people were really struggling. All eyes were on me and I had to have my public face on at all times. I did not want anybody to see any weakness in me. There were cameras here, there and everywhere. However, I could not show how much I was hurting. I felt I had to lead by example.

It was a very difficult first day. When I got back to the hotel I started physically shaking and was freezing cold. This lasted for almost an hour and I began to have doubts. I rang my brother and said, 'Neil, I can't do this, I don't know how I'm going to get through the next few days.' I was a physical and mental wreck, but Neil just reassured me and told me I could do it, for which I was grateful. Looking back I think my body was in shock and that is why I had reacted like that.

The first four days were supposed to be roughly 20 miles each, but it was more like 22, 28, 20, and then 23 on the fourth day. That was really difficult, it was both mentally and physically tough, because you set your mind on tackling 20-mile stretches, then suddenly another eight miles are thrown in on top of that. It is hard to come to terms with the extra bit – getting lost and doing more miles was the hardest part of the walk.

On the third night Steve Ball from the Rugby League Benevolent Fund organised for us to do a lap of the pitch at the Leeds v. Wigan play-off game. This was the first time we had met Steve. He was eager to make a good impression as we had chosen his Charity as one of the beneficiaries of the Steve Prescott Foundation. What an impression he made! Our 'Max and Paddy' motor home filled with all the walkers was greeted by Steve. He took it upon himself to back us into a tight parking space at the side of the B&B which he had arranged for us to stay in overnight. It went something like this, 'To me, to me, to me,' using his hand as a signal. We were all laughing as he sounded like the Chuckle Brothers.

Martin had been driving the van for a few days by this time and was aware of its size. He kept asking Steve, 'Are we ok above, is the height ok?'

Steve was confident in his response, 'Yes, yes!' Crash! Steve had failed to see the fire escape stairs attached to the building. This caused a big dent and a scratch to the roof canopy of both the motor home and also our profit margin for that event.

On leaving the motor home on our way to Headingley I had pain. I looked between my toes and saw bad blisters. The pus leaked over my hands. As I have no spleen, I have to be really careful about infections so I went to see the club doctor for some antibiotics.

We walked round the pitch at half time, receiving a fantastic reception from the crowd. I never thought I would hear the day that Leeds and Wigan fans would be singing my name. It was good for those walkers to get some recognition on Sky, as they had given up their time and put in a lot of effort. Too often it was made out to be all me and I felt embarrassed by that, so every time I spoke I made sure I mentioned them and stressed that it was a team effort.

Afterwards in the supporters bar, people approached to tell me their stories and experiences with cancer. It was very hard for me to listen and respond positively as it was all still very raw. Although I had received no counselling, I had found myself in an unqualified position of trying to help others. As time has passed this has become a lot easier for me but at that time I had only just began to speak about what I had been through and still found it intense.

Others would come up and say, 'My dad died with this type of cancer and my Nan died with that.' Conversations like that were tough, and it did affect my mental state, but we raised a lot of money and it was helping me to become stronger and face up to my situation.

The following day we back tracked to Featherstone and had to walk the journey to Leeds. The money raised on this leg was going to Brennan Rooney; he and his dad, Jamie, walked with us. Linzi and my eldest son Taylor had come over to see me and walked four or five miles with us. It was the same route I had done a few weeks earlier on another of Brennan Rooney's charity walks, so I thought it would be easy. But nothing is ever so straightforward and as we walked, we came to a roundabout; Martin's autoroute took us left. The week before we had gone straight on, but instead we went left, left and left again and ended up walking from Wakefield to the White Bear under the M62 via White Rose shopping centre.

We were all lost! We hadn't realised that there were two Dewsbury Roads in Leeds. I lay down on the floor and said, 'I can't go on any more.' I was physically wrecked. Taylor lay on the floor alongside me wondering what on earth I was doing. We trudged back to the vans – which dropped us off on the right track and we still had to walk another two miles to Headingley. I really hobbled them. That night I sat on the edge of the bath, cold water up to my shins, eating pizza. As I took the plasters off my blisters, pus just flowed out, it really frightened me.

On the Huddersfield leg we headed to the George Hotel, birthplace of rugby league, where Tommy Martyn presented his 1996 Challenge Cup winner's medal. How can you thank people like Tommy? He did two or three legs of the walk. Immediately afterwards, he sent me a text saying, 'Your bravery is unbelievable and you show great courage, whatever you do in future I will do it too.' And so he did – he is a good friend.

It was psychologically important for me to get over the Pennines into Lancashire. Once over there I knew a lot of my friends were going to be walking the Warrington to St Helens leg and I was looking forward to it. On the way through Thatto Heath, where I was born and brought up, my family were waiting for us and Koby was excited to see me (he had not walked with Linzi and Taylor because he was only one year old). Lots of people came out of the shops and houses talking to me and wishing us well. It was a good time but quite emotional. A lot of people came out of the Bird

I'th Hand pub and I walked down to the Knowsley Road ground chatting with Saints chairman Eamonn McManus.

The last day saw more than 50 of us set off from Leigh, including friends and family and my consultant and doctors from The Christie. When we got close to Old Trafford, Martin phoned to instruct me to stay a mile away from the stadium because Bill Arthur was ready with Sky, and Granada wanted to be there at the finish line. It was good that we stopped and regrouped because it allowed my little boy Taylor, who had walked that day, plus all the 11 full-time walkers to be at the front when we arrived. The others stayed towards the back giving us the privilege of walking in first.

We waited for Martin to come down the road in his Max and Paddy van and set off again for the home straight. I could sense the emotions starting to kick off inside everybody. It was really good and we could see the cameras in the distance waiting for us. When we actually got to Old Trafford I just completely broke down and started crying. I think it was relief that I had managed to do it and the sense of achievement of completing it felt like I had become close to all the other walkers. We shared the elation together. It was a very emotional moment and we cracked open the champagne under the Sir Matt Busby statue.

It was a great feeling and took me back to the days when we won the Challenge Cup. Martin and I hugged each other. He had organised it all and been there through thick and thin and we were both emotional over our achievement. Linzi gave me a hug too and then the 11 walkers had our pictures taken together. The Saints and Leeds fans who had assembled for the final began chanting my name which was quite embarrassing at the time. It was fantastic that we had all completed it together.

It was unfortunate that the RFL would only allow myself (I also took Taylor on with me), Mark Saunders, my consultant at The Christie, and Pete Stephenson, Rugby League Benevolent Fund beneficiary to go on to the pitch at Old Trafford for the cheque presentation. I was really upset by this as it was a group effort and I would not have got through it without the other team members, yet they had to watch from the stands. I would have loved for them to get the chance to go on the pitch and be in the spotlight. They deserved it.

Beforehand I did not realise how tough it was going to be, but try walking 28 miles and then doing it again the day after. You think to yourself, 'it is only walking', but it is tough, especially when that is all you are doing from 9.30am. It tested my head, my body and my legs. It was mentally tough doing this 11 days on the trot. We did what we set out to do which was to raise money. It was also an amazing response from my friends and family who were immense throughout. More than anything I wanted to show people that you can still do things despite being diagnosed with terminal cancer.

Looking back when I did the first Trans-Pennine walk I was not in great shape having just come off chemotherapy and my completion was largely down to the others getting me through it.

The second walk was different – and so was I. This time I was up at the front with Tommy Martyn, setting the pace all the way from Hull. Tommy had kept his word. He said he would do it all with me if I did it again and he did. Those who signed up expecting it to be the same pace as last time found it tougher. Admittedly, there were a few grumbles. They thought they had signed up for a three mile an hour pace but we were actually doing four mph. This was the determination kicking in. It was the turning point of getting mentally stronger and tougher.

It was a great start as many past and present players turned out to show their support, along with participants of the walk, new ones and ones from the previous year. The Benevolent Fund beneficiaries had also made the effort to join us on that day and I remember Martin announcing their presence in the pub in Hull beforehand. All the full-time walkers were delighted and inspired by their enthusiasm to get involved and overcome adversity. Martin asked for volunteers to assist with the wheelchairs and Tommy was first to hold his hand up. Jimmy Gittins and Paul Kilbride loved the involvement and the challenge. They were so inspired; they got a taste for the team spirit and camaraderie that they missed so much from their playing days, that they decided to come back the following day. It was great until we got to day four when Tommy realised how physically hard it was to push a wheelchair with the weight of the guys in them, along with monotonous miles of uphill and down dale roads in Yorkshire. It was mentally tough and it was agreed then that the pushing duties would be shared and we all took a turn.

We did have a laugh and it was the funny times that got us

through. We all had a bit of banter and we all learned to take the stick. As good as it was meeting all those people on the roadside and having a team of bucket collectors raising money for the Foundation, I knew when I reached Old Trafford that my next challenge would have to test me more. I needed that second walk to give me the appetite to go on to do more difficult challenges–walking was just not hard enough now.

18

A Marathon Effort

Although I have been a professional sportsman for most of my adult life, the London Marathon is right up there with one of the hardest things I have ever done. I have now done it three times. I first got the idea of taking part in December 2007 and I asked Martin Blondel to look in to whether it was possible to enter. The next thing I knew, he had secured me a place to run under The Christie banner and he was already booking hotel rooms.

Since my operation I had not done much distance running at all, in fact I had never done any long distance running so preparing for the marathon was just like starting out all over again. It meant I only had three months and 13 days to train for a 26 mile run, starting from scratch. I managed two runs at the end of December, but my time was hardly impressive – one mile in 11 minutes, which was really slow and both of my calves cramped up. I got off the machine at the gym and my brother said: 'Don't worry about it ... go away, come back tomorrow and you can build things up gradually.'

I came back, just before New Year and I did two miles in 24 minutes, but I was a hell of a way off 26 miles. For a spell it looked as though I would be running alone. I had spoken to Chris Joynt and I knew that he and Dave Lyon were doing the marathon through The Christie and they suggested we link-up. It was tough for Chris in the build-up. He was recovering from a broken ankle from playing rugby union which hampered his training somewhat, but he stuck at it.

I spoke to Terry O'Connor, who was into running and he expressed an interest in doing the London Marathon having done the Great North Run. We pulled a few strings and managed to get Terry a celebrity place and he became my running partner. Both Terry and I, along with Chris and Dave, started in the London Marathon 2008.

When I first started off I thought perhaps five hours would be a reasonable target. That's what I put down on the registration form as my estimated time. Apollo Perelini, my former team-mate and the Saints' conditioner, gave me a few extra sessions to freshen things up as part of my preparation. Apollo told me to just get on the bike and do a bit of cycling beforehand. His session was really hard as it turned out, something I had never really done before. It was only four-and-a-bit weeks before the marathon and it was the first time I had done leg weights. For the leg weights I did single leg squats on a ball with a weight round my neck ... I felt a bit like a shire horse. I carried on building up the distances but once I had got the 20-miler under my belt, that was it. I wasn't very confident, but there was no way I was doing any more long runs after that.

There were a few things to sort out before the actual run, however. The sheer complexity of the registration process did not help our preparations for the run at all. We went down on the train on Saturday morning, the day before the race. When you're out of your usual routine and you're struggling with your bags then it's easy to become dehydrated; you don't drink enough. We were on our feet all day, with two young kids in tow which didn't help preparation. People don't realise what is involved, I certainly didn't and I think that reason is why some people fail – poor preparation.

The weather was fine when we started and we set off at a reasonable pace. After the first mile in just under nine minutes we were down for 4 hours 40 minutes. We felt comfortable, so we kept on running at that pace. You certainly need energy boosts along the way and Terry and I had brought loads of these gel packs for our run. Terry had put them in his bum bag, but when I asked him for one, he unzipped the zipper and they had disappeared. We then had to rely on the good nature of the other runners and cadged what we could.

We were running nine minute miles and our half marathon time was 2 hours 3 minutes. It was going great, but unfortunately after 16 miles my left Achilles started getting a bit sore. Then I had twinges in my quads and I said to Terry that I needed to slow down. 'You'll be all right, just run through it,' he said. Then the pain started to get even worse. Both quads were cramped up and tight and I was running through the pain.

By the 19 mile mark my hamstrings were like clenched fists, so I had to stop and stretched straight away to try to loosen them. 'What a nightmare – of all the places to stop it would have to be right in front of the BBC cameras,' I thought.

After some more 'encouragement' from Terry we started again, but I was struggling and just waved at him to go on without me. It was horrendous. I had my phone with me and rang Linzi in tears because I thought I had ruined the whole marathon. She said, 'Keep going we're at the 22 mile mark. You can do it.' So for the next three miles I was grabbing every sweet I could from the sidelines. People were brilliant like that and I was sucking on a lollipop desperately trying to get something back in to my body. I was so pleased to see Linzi and the kids and ran over to give her a kiss. I don't know if the stuff I'd pumped into my body had started to work or if I had just got my running head back on and got rid of the demons in my mind.

Terry was struggling a bit himself by this point because we had started too fast, but I just thought, 'I've got to go for it,' so from 23 to 25.5 miles, I ran on my own and didn't stop once. I don't know how I did it, whether I blocked out the pain, but I was thinking, 'Finish, please finish!' My time was 4 hours 23 minutes with 1,000m to go and after picking up my pace up and weaving around numerous casualties I was in the home straight. However, just past Big Ben and with 400 metres to go both my groins cramped up badly. I couldn't move and had to stretch myself on the fence once more. I ran round the corner, past the finish line and stopped my watch ... 4 hours 32 minutes. I was gutted to miss my target by two minutes. I was so emotional at the time because I had been through hell but I couldn't have done any more.

People asked me beforehand, 'What's your aim in all of this?' I just wanted to complete it in the end ... but I had this niggling thing in the back of my mind. My dad did the same run in the early 90s and finished in 4 hours 30 minutes. I was just over two minutes away from success in this respect. Mind you, I have to say 'hands up!' My old fella's beaten me this time. He even slept in the back of a van the night before – there was no luxury hotel room for him.

The second time around I had learned some lessons from my first encounter and it helped that I was already in the capital on the Friday because I was picking up my MBE from Buckingham Palace. I was much fresher having been able to look after myself the day before, rather than being stressed rushing to register and spending hours on the train and tube.

I ran my second London Marathon with Mike Denning, the Steve Prescott Foundation chairman. Mike and I had trained together in St Helens over the dark and dingy winter training period, through the wind, rain and gloomy cold streets. On the day, we started off quicker than we had expected and when we reached the six-mile marker we were surprised at how well we were going. Mike was concerned he may be overdoing it and it could cost him later. We ran together up to a certain point, around the 10 mile mark. He didn't want to continue at that speed but he knew that I had to beat my previous time so he told me to crack on. Mike still says my boyish enthusiasm got the better of him.

From a personal point of view, I ran a much better race and only cramped up on the last mile and managed to beat my dad's time, which had been my target. We both successfully completed and we were also both elated with our times, 4hours 24minutes for me and 4 hours 41minutes for Mike, which was not bad for a fat kid! Well done Mike.

19

Catalan to Wembley

After completing the walks, I was ready to push the barriers further and we came up with plans that did just that, taking the challenge overseas, up mountains, down rivers and across the sea. The first of these challenges came up in August 2009 starting with a monster cycle ride from Perpignan, across the length of France to the English Channel; with further cycling back in England up to Uxbridge before paddling 24 miles up the River Thames in a dragon boat. We then undertook a half-marathon before entering Wembley Stadium with the match ball for the 2009 Challenge Cup Final. Such a big project required 'blue chip' sponsorship to the tune of £9,000, and we got that from Carnegie, Leeds, who were sponsoring the Challenge Cup at the time. Pete Stephenson and Jimmy Gittins, who were both seriously hurt playing rugby league, put themselves forward for the challenge. The look of satisfaction and achievement after their first session of dragon boat training in Liverpool said it all.

So Perpignan, the home of Catalan Dragons, was to be the starting point of a 13-day adventure which was a logistical nightmare to organise, plotting cycling routes, booking hotels and meals and making sure that the participants' health and safety was paramount, which proved to be a task in itself taking into account the different levels of ability and cycling speeds, which caused problems. We also had to deal with the French authorities. Initially, I wanted to row the English Channel but two weeks before it got under way the French authorities said no. Undeterred we threw in dragon boating down the Thames to make up for it.

Thirteen days is a long time to be away from home and family, but we got a good response from many businessmen and ex-players. Players got to know by word of mouth and our crew was quickly recruited. I was joined by ex players Anthony Sullivan, Paul Sculthorpe, Steve Hampson, Gary Connolly, Lee Jackson, Chris Joynt, Steve Hall, Chris Smith and Paul Barrow. *Sunday Mirror* rugby journalist and former Rochdale player David Burke also pitched in with his superb cycling skills, as did businessmen Mike Denning, Darren Harrison, Jimmy Rothwell, Barry Ford, John Kilgannon, Shaun Keenaghan, Richard Blowman, Paul Griffiths, John Mastin and Dave Gittins.

The support crew comprised of Will Young, Neil Coleman, Steve White, Martin Blondel, John Parry, Hugh Denning, Helen Pennington (physio), Becky Hinchcliffe, Alex Toms (camera crew) and Gary Brennand (support driver UK).

The itinerary gives a taste of what we were going to be up against.

- Day 1 Flight from Liverpool
- Day 2 Perpignan to Carcassonne
- Day 3 Carcassonne to Montauban
- Day 4 Montauban to Sarlat La Caneda
- Day 5 Sarlat La Caneda to Limoges
- Day 6 Limoges to Chateauroux
- Day 7 Chateauroux to Blois
- Day 8 Blois to Chartres
- Day 9 Chartres to Rouen
- Day 10 Rouen to Abberville
- Day 11 Abberville to Calais

There were plenty of incidents, accidents and comedy moments starting from the very beginning. We aimed to beat the worst of the baking heat on our first day, hence the 5.30am start from Perpignan, so we suggested a curfew at 11pm that night. However, a few of the lads – Scully, Gary Connolly, Paul Barrow and John Kilgannon – came in during the early hours, and as a result some were still intoxicated when they were pumping their tyres up. This wasn't safe but we are a charity, not their minders. It was totally up to them. I can understand them wanting to have a good time and enjoy the trip as well as putting in the hard work on the challenge.

The preparation wasn't ideal and it began to show on some of the participants. John Killgannon could hardly ride and Paul Barrow came off his bike two miles into the day's 100 mile journey. We also got lost going from our hotel to Catalans stadium so we and ended up doing extra mileage around the town. It was a bad start! Although we aimed to avoid the soaring temperatures, it was inevitable from the start we had that it would catch up with us.

Initially, we tried to stay in one group but it was difficult due to the varying levels of ability among the cyclists. It was a logistical nightmare for the people in vans and cars who were supporting us, as everybody was spread out over miles. It was tough and during the first day, we endured quite a mountainous climb in 40 degree heat. It was the first time we hit a major hill – John Kilgannon cracked first and was thrown in the van and driven up the hill. But there was no way I was quitting, that's not my style. I was doing every single mile without help.

After the first day we had an emergency meeting and decided we had lost control cycling in one big group, I was a bit upset because I envisioned us all cycling together but that was not possible so we came up with a contingency to split into three groups – top, middle and bottom. As a rule Team Carbon, the elite cyclists, just flew off and had their feet up by 1pm. They comprised David Burke, Paul Sculthorpe, former Great Britain and Wigan full back Steve Hampson and ex-Saints wing Steve Hall among others. They had done a lot of training and were good cyclists so we let them get on with it with absolutely no resentment. They thoroughly deserved the extra rest they gained at the end of the day and I just wished I could have been up there with them, but it was out of my league.

My group, the middle one, got better as cyclists as the challenge progressed and we even came up behind Team Carbon on one occasion and shot past them – you should have seen their faces. It was a bit of fun and banter although we tried to make sure the third group was not disheartened so we asked some of the elite cyclists to go with them to give them a boost. However, that did backfire when we put Gary Connolly into group three. He had them bombing in the water park instead of cycling, so instead of getting back to base at 5pm they arrived at more like 7pm.

It was great fun and the banter helped us get through what was a tough challenge. Former Saints skipper Chris Joynt came up with a competition to do tasks along the way, like taking obscure pictures. So they had shots of us squashed in a phone box, on the church altar, packed in a mini and cycling naked. It was great fun, became an added challenge and it passed the day.

Joynty was full of one-liners throughout the duration of the challenge. He is a really funny guy with a dry sense of humour. You could tell he could have been in the top group of cyclists had he wished, but he wanted to enjoy the experience and looked after the group as a whole. It was, I suppose, just like the way he used to look after his Saints team when he was captain. He is a great bloke and I have huge respect for him.

To add to the enjoyment and fun there was a jersey presentation every night. The yellow jersey was given to an inspirational figure of that day, while a pink one was awarded if you had been a letdown or if you'd done something comical.

On the whole the jerseys provided a cracking laugh with John Kilgannon getting the pink jersey most days. I came very close to getting it one day after letting the frustration of a hard day's cycle get the better of me. On arrival at one of the hotels, a key was handed to me for the room I was sharing with Steve White. So off we went, carrying our equipment and heavy bags up to the fourth floor as we couldn't fit in the lift, only to find somebody else was actually staying in that room. So back down to reception we went with all our kit and lo and behold exactly the same thing happened to us.

Third time lucky I thought as I was handed yet another key and promised this room would be vacant. It was but it was a double bed and there was no way I was spooning with Ste and I was fuming. I stormed back down the flights of stairs to the reception and demanded that this was sorted as I was not lugging my belongings up anymore unless it was correct. The receptionist told me that I would have to wait 10 minutes whilst she sorted things out. My reply to her was, 'Ok then I'll wait right here.' I proceeded to sit down right on the spot in the middle of reception, with my arms and legs folded like a spoilt little school boy. I admit I spat my dummy out and looking back it is quite embarrassing. I did take some stick for it but it worked and within minutes I was given the correct room key. The rest of the lads were in fits of laughter seeing me throw a small tantrum like that, but I suppose I'm only human.

It was not all a joke – and Chris Smith took it on himself to be finesmaster to help keep discipline. If you were one minute late getting up or going down for dinner you had to settle up with Smiggy. People did not want to get fined, but if he said you were fined you were fined, there was no appeal. I was only fined once during the trip. It was on day four at Sarlat La Caneda and I wouldn't have minded so much if it was my fault, but I suppose I can't say that as I am responsible for myself. I was still rooming with Ste White and he is a great lad. He always set his alarm so that we were up in plenty of time and we were both pretty organised, getting our gear ready each night for the next day's cycling. That night we all went out for a meal. Ste being Ste wanted to stay out, socialise and have a beer. I knew how my body was feeling and with a tough day the next day I wanted to get myself a good night's sleep, so I left him to it with the rest of the lads. I got back to my room, laid out all my cycling gear, got my bag sorted for the following day and got my head down.

The hours seemed to fly by and when I heard a noise and realised it was Ste having a shower I forced myself to get out of bed, wishing I had an extra few hours, and began to get dressed into my full kit, socks, shoes, my cycling bib shorts, shirt and gloves. When Ste emerged from the shower looking a bit worse for wear he looked surprised to see me up in full gear and asked, 'What are you doing? It's 3am!' To add to the frustrations Ste then forgot to set the alarm which he had done daily up to this point. We were 30 minutes late the next morning going down for breakfast, and were welcomed by the cheers and amusement of the other lads. I was irate at the thought of a 50 Euro fine and Ste felt guilty because he didn't like to let anyone down. With the rush, Ste didn't have time to do his usual morning grooming and with his lack of sleep and copious beers, he looked rough and his hair was sticking up all over the place which earned him the nickname 'Ken Dodd'. I soon forgave him and still thought the fine system was what was needed. The system raised an additional £600 for the Foundation.

David Burke was an absolute gentleman, and he was brilliant cycling despite having a bike that seemed very old fashioned. It worked for him, though. He wanted to be involved in the challenge and relished being in Team Carbon. In fact he wanted more, and on day three of the challenge he asked if he could cycle another 15 miles because he had spotted a lake he wanted to swim in. David did tell me that it was a fair but hard tackle from my dad that ended his career as a player in the late 1970s when he was in the Blackpool team against Salford.

We were joined on the challenge by Jimmy Gittins and Pete Stephenson who did their cycling on a quad bike, along with their own support crew. Jimmy and Pete are former amateur rugby league players who broke their necks playing the game. Seeing them doing it was fantastic, but they had special needs given their disabilities. We gave their support staff some leeway to take part in the challenge themselves – but it did cause some issues, particularly when the duo got lost on their quad bike and on one occasion were stopped by the police. They are both fantastic ambassadors for the game of Rugby League and it takes a lot of courage and bravery to do the events and challenges they take on. I admire them both so much and am proud that they participate and push themselves for the Charity.

After the cycling legs were done, we had to face the dragon boats for 24 miles down the River Thames, where the weather was slightly mixed; one minute we were shivering because it was raining and the next minute we were too warm because the sun would be cracking the flags. St Helens comedian Johnny Vegas lifted the spirits when he turned up on a motorbike taxi, carrying a pint of Guinness, and joined us in the boat for a leg down the river. Dragon boating sounds like a quaint little pastime but it was hard work travelling from Windsor to Teddington Lock. We were all paddling and it took 11 hours, so people were tired and then we had to run a half marathon the following day. Once again some of the lads prepared differently for that last leg. Gary Connolly and Paul Barrow went for a night on the town and came sneaking in, almost commando style across the floor, past me and Linzi whilst we were having breakfast in the hotel. Paul basically came in, put his shorts on and ran 13 miles, while Gary simply took to his bed. So having done all of France, the dragon boating and painfully hard work for 13 days, Gary decided not to complete the challenge on the last day. He had done what he wanted to do. It wasn't because he had been on the beer but because all through the event he had been saying that running wasn't for him with his bad knee – fair play to him.

Our half marathon run from RAF Uxbridge to Wembley Stadium was a bit of a shambles. Unbelievably, having got through from France and all the other trials and tribulations, it all went tits up on the last leg. We all ended up running in different directions. The run itself was horrendous because our quads were shot to bits from the cycling. Our group ran into Wembley Stadium together and I put the ball on the centre spot and then we did a lap of honour. It was a good sense of achievement for the 24 of us who did that challenge. I was conscious that I wanted it to be about what we had done as group; I did not want it to be just about me. It did feel a little bit like I was hogging the limelight when I put the ball on the centre spot, surrounded by photographers.

One of the positive aspects of setting up these challenges, be it the cycling, boxing or rugby, is that it allows me and some of the lads I've played with to experience the buzz of being part of a team again. Any retired sports professional will tell you that it is hard to switch off from a competitive environment if you have been trained to be competitive from a very young age. I think that is one of the reasons people sign up and make big sacrifices to do these things with me – they want to give themselves another challenge and enjoy some of the team banter.

Martin does his best to get things sorted for those taking part, even if he gets his protein and potassium mixed up, but he has had to learn how to be around a sporting environment. We also have to watch the budget because what we spend obviously comes out of what we give over at the end of the event. Going to France was a massive outlay and we did get a lot of stick about those costs, but at the end of day we still raised £32,000 profit for the Charities.

People don't realise how difficult events are to organise for a small charity. The process involves route planning, sorting out the bikes and spares, ensuring everyone's safety, booking accommodation and sorting the food. I, among others, did my fair share of moaning on some challenges, especially about the food but deep down I know how hard it is and the support always give 100 per cent to make sure we are all okay.

20

Keep on Running

If you think running one marathon is tough, think about tackling five of them in a row, back-to-back, including four of them across the Pennines in damn awful weather conditions. The plan was to run, not walk, from Hull to Old Trafford, again ahead of the 2010 Super League Grand Final. The last marathon was to be staged on treadmills in the Engage Fanzone outside the Theatre of Dreams, giving fans, celebrities and friends a chance to get involved in the challenge on the final day.

This was another big challenge; just the sort that I was looking for, even though Martin thought it was going to be too much for me and kept telling me so. To be fair to Martin, he was right, it was too hard – but I had an incident on the first day that made it even tougher.

It was my idea to run from Hull to Old Trafford, taking the event up a significant few notches from the Trans-Pennine walks. I wanted to show people that this was an 'extreme event' and it got some good publicity. Unfortunately, I didn't know how to train for this one so it came to a point where I simply left it. The plan was to run six miles and then take a break, and then run another six miles and so on. It did not work because I never felt the benefit of stopping and realised it was probably easier to keep on running.

We ran 30 miles on the first day – but after the first six miles we stopped to get some food to boost our energy levels. Ridiculously, thinking about it, I accepted the option of bananas.

Due to my ileostomy and the way I now digest food, all fruit is banned from my diet, but I knew at this time I had a long way to go and I needed to get some energy from somewhere to help get me to the end of the first day. Martin, who was always thinking about the charity profits, decided to buy a load of green bananas so they would last the whole challenge and not go bad. I should have known that unripe bananas of all things would cause me trouble. In normal circumstances I would have stayed well clear but the daunting task ahead clouded my judgement.

With ten miles to go I was in absolute agony. I knew that the pain I was experiencing was an obstruction of the bowel. On quite a number of occasions I have been admitted to hospital when under an obstruction and it is a matter of waiting until it clears. The suffering I endure when they strike is torture. The number is in double figures now where I have had to be kept in hospital and put on morphine while my body gets rid of the obstructions in my bowel. I kept telling myself this wasn't happening and the pain would reside but with five miles to go, I turned to Nicky Reid, my close friend, who I was running alongside, and said, 'I'm going to be in hospital tonight.' I completed the day but went straight to bed, praying that the blockage would relieve itself. I was in torment but had no strong pain killers. Martin panicked when he saw how bad I was and realised I wouldn't be continuing with the challenge and it was only the end of day one. Whilst Martin was trying to put a plan B in to action, phoning around other ex-players who had helped the charity in the past, I just wanted to be left alone in my room!

Basically, I did it the hard way by spewing up bile, getting everything out of my system, spending the night on the bathroom floor with a pillow and a paracetamol. Obviously it meant I had no sleep and there was nothing left in my body. How was I going to run when I couldn't even pack my own belongings?

All the participants came to my room to tell me they would get through the day without me, and when they saw how bad I was it was confirmed to them that they would have to. I was devastated because I felt like I was letting them all down. How could I ask them to put their bodies through the next 30 miles if I wasn't doing it myself?

Usually, when this strikes, it takes me two or three days in hospital and then a week to recover from the trauma at home. That's

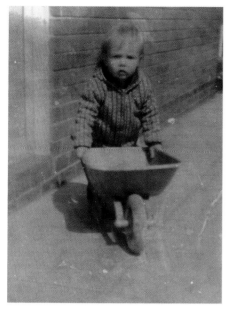

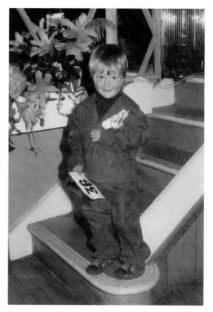

Pushing a wheelbarrow at
home, aged 2

Fancy dress competition – me
as The Six Million Dollar Man!

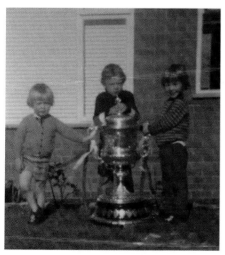

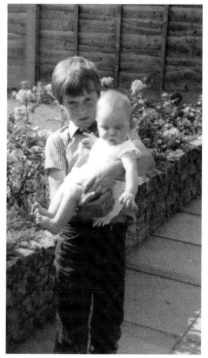

Proudly stood with the
Championship trophy won by
my dad at Salford in 1976

Holding my baby sister Suzanne
in our back garden in Nutgrove

Me with my football cups, with brother Neil and sister Suzanne

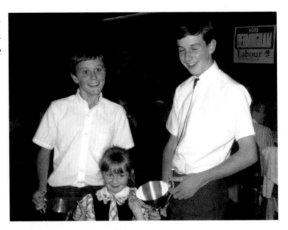

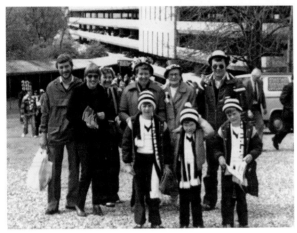

Supporting my dad – and Widnes – with family at Wembley in 1981

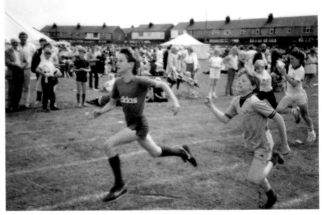

Winning the sprint at the St Austin's field day in 1985

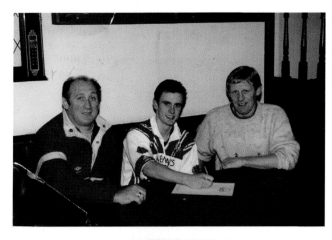

Signing for Saints watched by Eric Chisnall and my dad Eric in November 1992

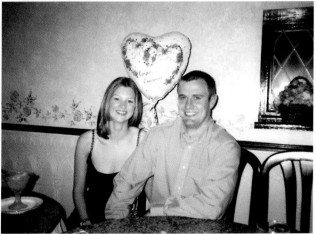

Myself and Linzi on the night of our engagement at Quattros in 1997

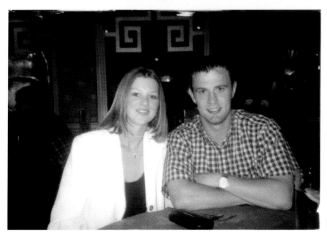

Celebrating with Linzi on her 21st birthday

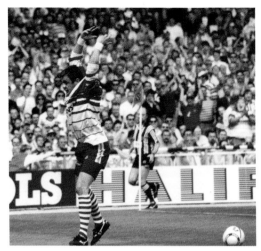
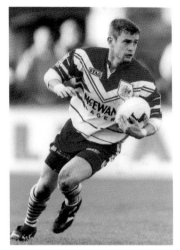

Celebrating one of my two tries at
Wembley in 1996

On the attack for Saints
in 1996

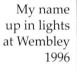

My name
up in lights
at Wembley
1996

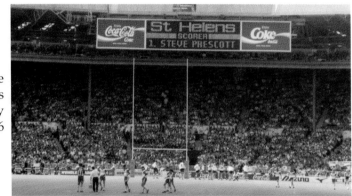

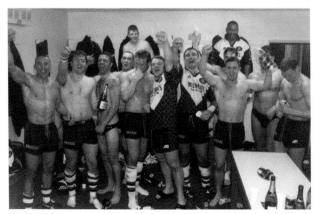

We're going to
Wembley! The
Saints dressing
room after the 1997
Challenge Cup
semi-final win over
Salford at Central
Park

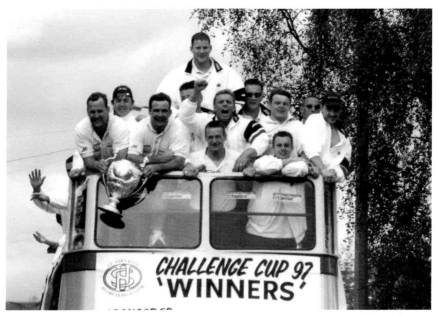

Wembley winners again! 1997 homecoming

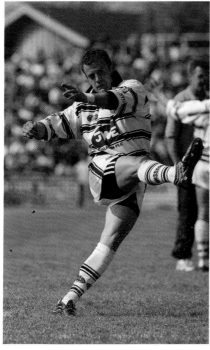

Kicking a goal for Hull FC

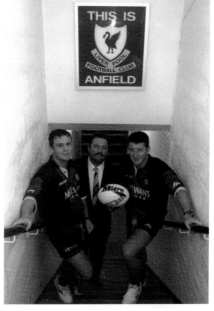

With coach Shaun McRae and
Julian O'Neill promoting Saints'
game at Anfield in 1997

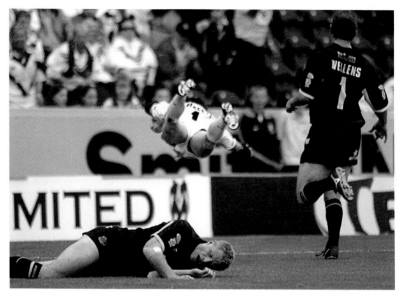

Flying in for a try, leaving Darren Albert on the floor
© *RLPhotos.com*

Life was unpredictable at Wakefield
© *RLPhotos.com*

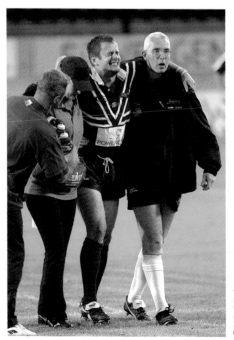

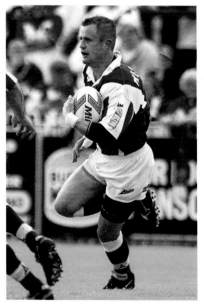

Agony! Breaking my knee cap in what would be my last ever professional game in July 2003
© *RLPhotos.com*

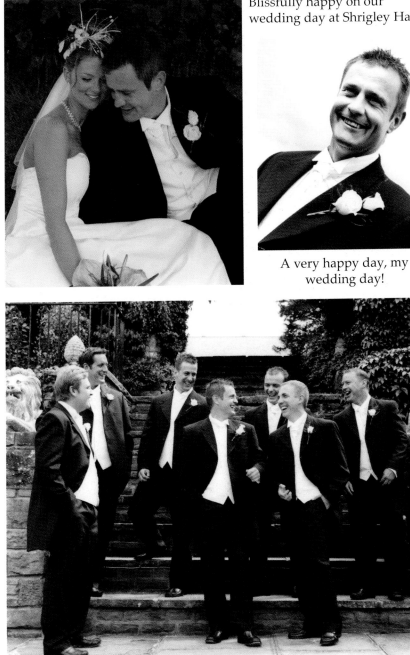

Blissfully happy on our wedding day at Shrigley Hall

A very happy day, my wedding day!

With my pals Paul Wright, Paul Barrow, brother Neil, myself, John Riley, best man Mike Ford and Mike Simmons at my wedding at Shrigley Hall

At home with new-born Koby, just
days after my diagnosis

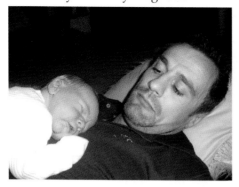

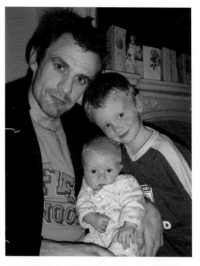

Myself, Taylor and Koby on the eve of
my big operation in Basingstoke

With Stuart
Fielden and Lee
Radford after the
Rumble on the
Humber in 2007

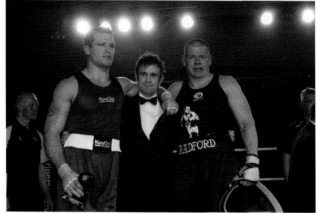

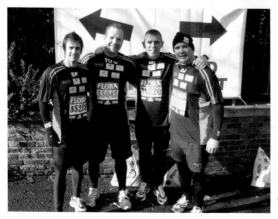

With Terry O'Connor,
Dave Lyon and Chris
Joynt after the 2008
London Marathon

At home with Koby,
Taylor and Linzi

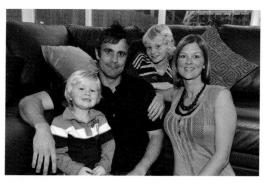

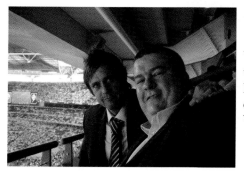

Watching the Cup Final
with my good friend
Martin Blondel as guests
of Phil Clarke in a box at
Wembley in 2007

Myself and good friend Mike
Denning, using bin bags to
sneak in to the starting line
together ahead of the 2010
London Marathon

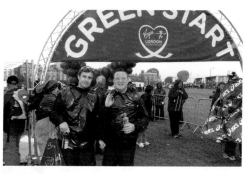

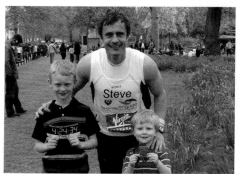

With my boys Taylor and
Koby in Hyde Park after the
2010 London Marathon

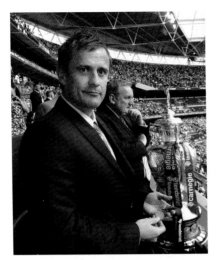

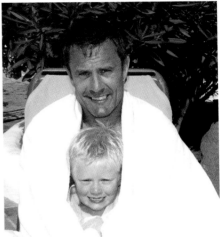

Waiting to present the Challenge
Cup at Wembley in 2010

Me and Koby by the pool on
holiday

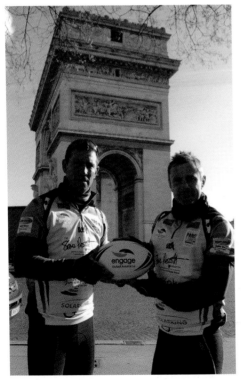

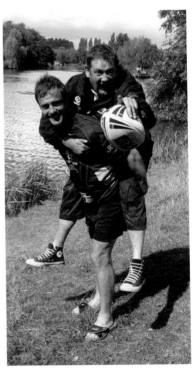

With Paul Sculthorpe in Paris during
the Paris to London Challenge

Giving Johnny Vegas a piggy
back during the dragon boating
challenge on the Thames

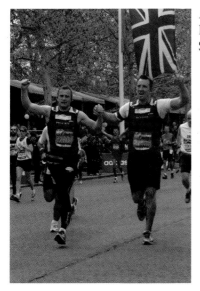

A personal best! Crossing the finishing line of the 2012 London Marathon with Scully – we smashed it together!

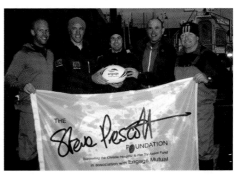

Myself and fellow crew Steve Hall, Scully, Chris Joynt and Bernard Dwyer just ahead of rowing the Channel

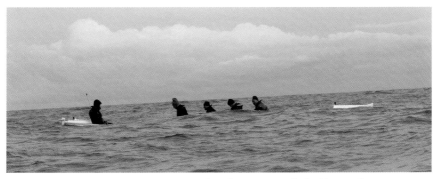

Five men in a boat on the choppy English Channel

Making Taylor and Koby laugh at the hotel in Dubai in 2012

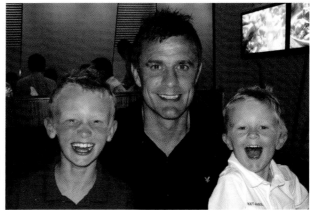

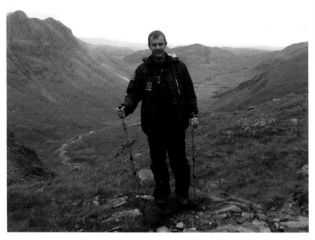

Climbing Scafell
Pike during the
Lands End to John
O'Groats Challenge

The full crew
at the top of
Snowdon –
the first of
three peaks
cracked!

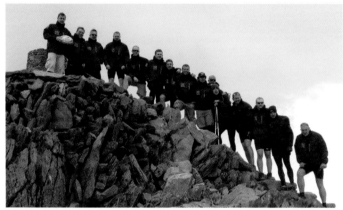

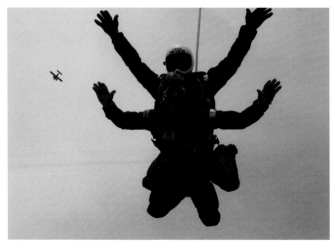

Adrenalin rush!
Skydiving
with the Red
Devils at Langar
Airfield near
Nottingham in
June 2010

Myself, Linzi, Taylor and Koby in Lanzarote in 2010

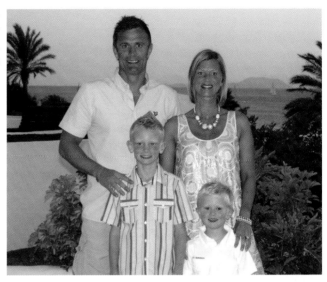

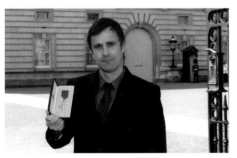

Collecting my MBE from Buckingham Palace

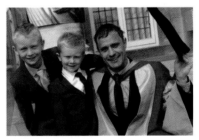

With my boys Taylor and Koby during my graduation ceremony at Hull University

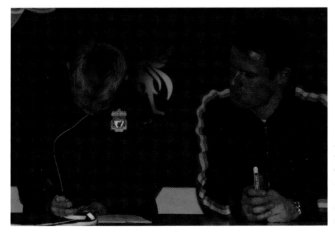

A proud day watching Taylor sign for Liverpool FC alongside Jamie Carragher

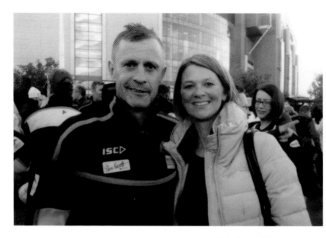

Me and Linzi
outside Old
Trafford after
the October 2012
challenge

Chemotherapy
at The Christie in
November 2012

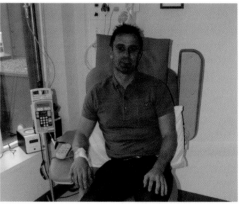

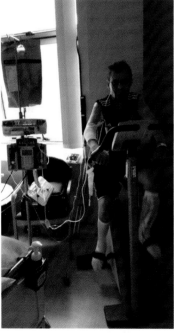

Getting in shape for the
battle ahead – on my bike
at the hospital in Oxford in
August 2013

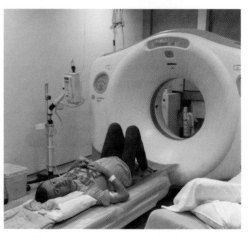

Undergoing a scan at Oxford in
September 2013

In intensive care at The Churchill Hospital, Oxford on October 4, 2013

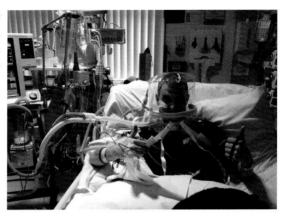

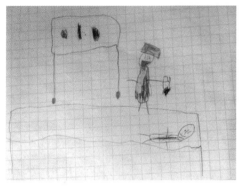

Koby's sketch of what my operation would look like – with surgeon Anil holding the knife

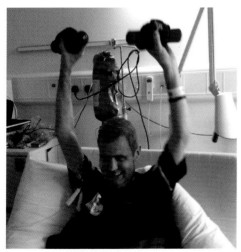

Not giving up! Doing weights in hospital on October 10, just days before the transplant

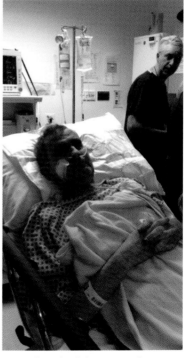

Ahead of the transplant

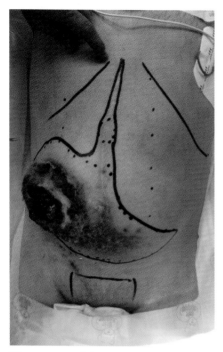

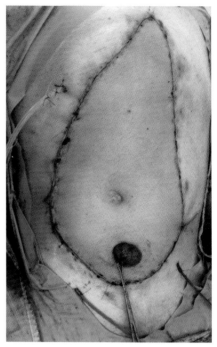

The extent of the tumour just before my final operation

The finished job after the transplant

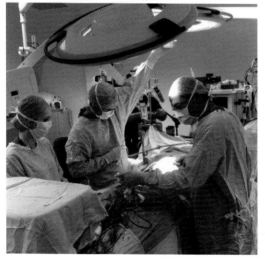

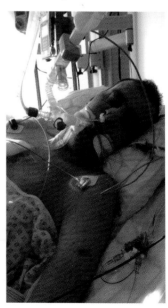

Mr Anil Vaidya and Mr Henk Giele conducting the transplant at Oxford

After the transplant

why I didn't take Martin's advice and go into hospital because I knew it would have meant the challenge was over. Martin was saying they were going to cancel it. To make the morning even more problematic, Sky Sports' Fraser Dainton had travelled over to do a piece with me about the event and how I inspire people with cancer to carry on. Instead, Mike Denning had to front up to the camera and inform them what was going on.

Martin pleaded to take me to hospital that morning but instead I had a cup of tea, piece of toast and an hour's sleep and then I insisted on getting in the car to catch up the other lads. Although I was as green as the Incredible Hulk, with nothing left in my body, fortunately the obstruction had cleared. My mind was made up to attempt to get on the road again slow-trotting the last five miles to Headingley with a very inflamed bowel and a distended, tender abdomen.

We stayed in Leeds that evening; I had a good night's sleep which set me up nicely to run the third day to Huddersfield. There was a real sense of achievement on my part to get through day three, but there were still tough days ahead. That fourth day included an 11-mile climb to the top of the Pennines over Saddleworth Moor. I was in a fragile state and when we got to the other side there was wind, hail, rain and fog. We stopped at a pub for a warm, a cup of soup and a change of clothing. Looking out of the window it looked like a scene from the *Wizard of Oz*, with a tornado blowing through – all that was missing was the witch on a bike with a broomstick.

We got through it and were met at Old Trafford by Sky, BBC and Granada. I was so upset, though, because I couldn't believe I had got to the end. It was sheer relief, elation and emotion pouring out of me. I had completed my part of yet another gruelling challenge. All that was left was day five, which was down to others to complete. Fans, joined by Sky journalist Angela Powers, England coach Steve McNamara, Terry O'Connor, Martin Offiah MBE, Shaun Briscoe, Ben Thaler, who ran the quickest mile, my consultant, Mark Saunders, Engage employees and Sid the Pig with my eldest son, Taylor, fittingly, running the very last mile. That made me proud.

Out of the five full-time runners that started, David Burke and Tony Barrow were the only ones to complete every single mile. It was more than four marathons – with a couple of 30-milers in there. Tony had a day where he struggled, but I couldn't believe Burkey was so strong– especially given his age – he was unbelievably fit.

People don't realise how tough it is doing things like this, especially with my condition. This is one of the reasons I wanted to write a book so people can get an insight into the truth. Some people think I am all right now, especially when they see me smiling in the papers and completing physically enduring challenges, but my body is different and I have to cope with that on a day to day basis. It was only on this challenge that my friends actually witnessed what I go through as even they didn't realise the extent of the complications I experience. They were upset to see me that way and it made me understand what Linzi must go through seeing me suffer as it is only her that usually sees me that way.

The fact that I got back on the road and completed the event showed me how much stronger I had become since the first walk and how much I had progressed. It showed I had more to give and the more extreme the better.

Martin asked me about doing another walk because they were popular with the public and very inclusive – but I wanted to challenge myself more. As a foundation we realised we had to be eye-catching, adventurous and take it to another level – we were now doing extreme challenges.

They say that variety is the spice of life – so again it was something different for the next big challenge. We strayed from the rugby league heartlands to take up Chris Joynt's earlier suggestion that we should cycle from Land's End to John O'Groats – the daddy of all domestic challenges. That idea had lingered on our minds for a few years but when I was training for my second London Marathon, one of the Foundation's committee members, Steve White, cycled LEJOG in an incredible 10 days with his Bardon work colleagues, in aid of the Charity.

The problem was he completed it successfully ... so we had to make our challenge tougher. The 15 of us cycled the full route in nine days and then we added in climbing the highest peaks of Wales, England and Scotland en route. It was probably insane. It was something different, new and really difficult. There were also 150 more miles than the End to End Bardon challenge as well as the three climbs.

Looking back I did not do nearly enough training for LEJOG and found the whole event really difficult from start to finish. You learn from your mistakes and my biggest one on this occasion was neither being measured up nor set up properly for my new bike. So from day one until the last day I suffered pain from the right knee that I had damaged and which ended my playing career. On this route you don't get broken in gently. Day one was such a massive shock to the system as we clocked 146 miles including a mammoth 10,000ft climb on a baking hot day. To put that into some context, that was a bigger climb than we did in the whole of France during the Carnegie Challenge. Put it this way, on day one we had only 40 miles on the clock and I was ready for quitting. When we reached our first stop of the day in Cornwall, Martin declared, 'When in Rome ...' and we had to get a Cornish pasty. It was the worst thing we could have eaten – imagine having to get on a bike after wolfing one of those big things down. It absolutely battered me with indigestion for the rest of the day.

We had a late start at 8am so it meant we did not get off our bikes until 10pm, which brought problems we had not legislated for ... the dark. We had not thought about putting lights on our bikes, so late in the day the police began taking an interest in us. With lights being a problem on the bikes and the days being longer than originally anticipated, we had to start earlier on subsequent days.

It was chaos on that first day because the groups had split into two, some got lost and others suffered punctures. I felt sorry for a Saints fan called Sharon Boulton, who waited hours with her family to greet us at the end of that first day. By the time we arrived at the end point in Exeter we were well behind schedule and all she got in return for her wait was a quick hello from an exhausted bunch of cyclists. From the outset we had stressed the need to eat the right food and the importance of getting the right nutrition to sustain us, but by 10pm, after 146 miles in the scorching heat, that went out of the window and it was a quick pizza delivery in the hotel room before retiring for the night ready for day two.

Cornwall was a tough county to start with and there were many more challenging days to follow. There were times during this event that I was mentally drained, more so than on any other challenge I had done to date. In fact I can remember when I was interviewed on the radio, I burst into tears, which is not like me but that is how it affected me. I have never been so emotional but I was dealing with my illness and my knee and a really gruelling schedule. I was totally exhausted and at the end of each day I questioned myself as to whether I would complete the next day. It did not get easier and the third day saw a 5.30am start, cycling 107 miles and then a four hour climb of Snowdon – it was a good mountain to start with and some of us got to see our families on that day in Llangollen. They also met up with us later in the day at the start of the climb. It was a great boost for me to have my two boys there and I was so proud to see Taylor, who was 10 years old, successfully climb to the summit with us. Linzi took Koby up to the top of the mountain on the train so they could congratulate us when we reached the top. We got the opportunity to pass a rugby ball around at the summit and have a bit of fun before the descent.

We were not without any hiccups on this challenge – not just because Hughie Denning, who was one of the support team, never really got the hang of the Sat Nav. Hughie is 76 and like a dad to everyone. We all have huge respect for him and love having him around. He is Irish through and through and we always have banter with him as not many get the hang of his accent until they've been around him for a few days. His only downfall is that he is not really technically minded. Every day he would get lost – and for some reason, Jon Neill and I continually put our faith in him. We also put our bags with spare clothes and snacks with him for the day – which was a huge mistake, especially as my bag contained all my tablets. One day I said, 'Hey Hughie, is it worth putting my bag in your car ... will I see it again today?'

One of the boys had hit a bollard on the Severn Bridge, doing a full somersault over the handle bars and damaging his bike in the process. Martin asked Hughie to make his way over quickly – his Sat Nav was saying he was only six miles away. After about 20 minutes Martin rang Hughie again to ask where he was and Hughie told him he was still heading for the bridge and the Sat Nav said there were 23 miles to go. Quick wittedly, Martin asked him, 'What bloody bridge are you heading for – Runcorn Bridge?

There were other crashes with Neil Harmon, the former Leeds and Warrington prop who I had toured with, coming off his bike and falling into the road smashing his helmet, just missing a lorry. Ste Hall, too, had a bad accident coming through Lancaster. He ended up with a massive graze down his hip and arms and he ripped all his expensive cycling clothing, which he was more bothered about than the injuries he had sustained. Then there was Nigel Johnston, a business colleague of my good friend Paul Barrow, who did the last four days with a bad injury after falling off his bike. The support team were concerned about him cycling with one arm and asked him to take some time in the support vehicle but he really wanted to complete the challenge. As it turned out, when he got home he went for an x-ray which confirmed he had actually broken a bone.

We reached the second mountain in Cumbria on day five after a 6.45am start from Lancaster. The weather was horrendous. It was so bad that the guide wasn't sure whether or not we would make it to the top. It took us six-and-and half hours to scale Scafell and when we came down we still had 48 miles to cycle. It was the toughest climb of the three, one with much more difficult terrain, involving jumping from boulder to boulder near the top. We ended the day at 9.45pm that night after a gruelling 14 hour ordeal.

The day after we had 142 miles from Penrith to Dunbarton to complete and I thought it was going to get the better of me. On the way we all stopped exhausted and lay on the lay-by of a busy Scottish road. It had got to the point of the challenge were we were looking for a plan B. People were talking about not being able to finish as we still had another 70 miles to go. We decided to have a committee meeting at the side of the road where we decided we needed to pick everyone up and get each other through. We did and two days later Ben Nevis was in front of us and we made good use of ice treatment, anti-inflammatories and pain killers. We soldiered on and got through it despite being in so much pain. I was in tears pushing down on the pedal, but one or two of the others stayed with me to help me along.

We hired a guide for Ben Nevis which was costly but worthwhile and he immediately recommended we strip off to our skins and take off our heavy clothes. He was very serious and professional, so straight away we thought we would wind him up by sending over Hughie Denning wearing a climbing rucksack, walking poles, sandals and socks. The guide looked at him and in disbelief said, 'Are you doing it in those sandals?' To which Hughie replied: 'If they were good enough for Jesus to walk to Calvary then they are good enough for me.' Hughie, of course, stayed in the van.

The guide was fantastic and given it was nearly 30 degrees going up it was right for us to take the heavy clothes off as he recommended. We looked a right sight going up – all I had on was a compression top and compression tights. The guide was constantly watching my every move. My knee was causing me a lot of trouble and after about an hour into the climb he stopped me and told me to make a decision as I was limping so badly – he put it to me that I should turn around and go back down – but I had to get to the top. Ben Nevis is the most enjoyable mountain you can climb. We still had 86 miles to do after descending the mountain. The conditions were awful, everyone was shattered, people were lost and the Sat Nav added another 10 miles on to our journey.

I really struggled with the whole event. For the first time it raised doubts in my mind as to whether illness had kicked in and whether I was getting weaker. On the other hand the events were getting much harder. It was by far the hardest event I had done at that point – causing so much pain and mental torture but ironically, the last day was the best day for cycling for me and I felt stronger than I had the whole way through.

Crossing the finishing line at John O'Groats was extremely emotional and to do this challenge in nine days was an unbelievable achievement. The big Cumbrian prop, Jon Neill, who I played with at Saints, helped me a great deal on this challenge. For the last two days I hid in behind big Jon which benefited me greatly, shielding me from the wind. Apparently, if you tuck yourself behind another rider, you use 30 per cent less energy. Jon is such a strong rider, with a huge frame, and I would have really struggled to make it home without that support. I can't thank him enough. Paul Stevens also helped me out greatly. He was one of those riders who was more bothered about getting me and the rest of the group through than his own self preservation and that meant a lot to me.

LEJOG raised over £20k for the charity and it was an unforgettable experience for all those who completed it.

We should have had a leisurely drive back – but Martin had agreed for me to appear on *Granada Reports* at 6pm after taking a call from Mike Hall that morning. Granada wanted me live in the studio so James Ogden along with Martin and I flew down the motorway in the support car, being quite rude to everyone who was in our way – without thinking about all the sponsors' stickers on the car. We arrived with two minutes to spare, not soon enough for Martin who ended up having a wee in the Granada studios car park. I had packed all my belongings previous to the phone call and my bag was on the support van. It wasn't until half way there I realised what I looked like. I hadn't had a shave, had bags under my eyes and was wearing flip flops as my feet were so sore. I didn't, for one minute, think that the camera man would pan out and show my footwear to the region. My wife was mortified. She had phone calls from her friends in fits of laughter as they knew she would be proud but wishing she had dressed me.

There is always doubt in my mind when I complete a challenge that I won't be able to do any more and that will be my last. As time goes on I suppose the disease progresses too. After LEJOG Martin thought I had reached that point and I had had enough. A short time afterwards I had recovered and I turned to him and asked, 'What are we doing next?'

21

Pride in St Helens

I am proud of St Helens – the town I was born and brought up in but I am not blind to some of the problems it now faces. As a town St Helens gets a little bit left behind at times. The borough has struggled to come to terms with industrial decline after the mines closed down, with Beechams gone and Pilkington Glass employing nowhere near the numbers it used to. And in stark contrast to neighbouring Liverpool, Warrington, Wigan and Widnes the leisure and retail sector has not really taken off. We can sit back and moan about what we have and have not got as a town, but I would rather to do something more constructive as well as doing something that celebrates the considerable achievements of our townsfolk.

Setting up the St Helens 10K, the Pride of St Helens Awards and even the sporty fun days at Taylor Park are all part of my desire to do something positive for my home town. I would like to think, given the numbers now turning out, that the events have filled a void.

Plenty of other towns have half marathons and that is why I wanted to establish one in St Helens. Some will find it strange, especially given I hated long-distance running with a passion as a player. Fun and running were never words that sat easily together for me. The Foundation has now organised three 10K road runs, with the second one being even bigger and better than the maiden one and the third race topping that. Of course there were problems sorting it out and the rules and stipulations from the council are hard to deal with – sometimes mind-bogglingly confusing. In fact, all we got from the local authority to assist us for the first 10K was a map of the route. Logistically, it is a frightening thing to organise – the Foundation is only a small organisation but now we have so many people running.

The events are getting bigger but there are only a few of us looking after them. We never get any funding or discount; there is no special dispensation for us as a charity, in fact in the first year we were even billed a considerable amount for having some bollards removed and replaced because they had stipulated we could not use a certain road.

I understand it is difficult for the council these days and local authorities are having money taken off them left, right and centre. However, it is really difficult for us as a small charity because we always seem to be battling against some form of red tape. One of the problems we have encountered has been if we change the course slightly we have to pay, and we ended up paying another £1,500 in the third race because we moved the course. At times we end up wondering why we bother. But we can see past that to the big picture of the benefit we are bringing by putting on activities here. That said, in the first ever 10K run there was one complaint delivered personally by a disgruntled member of the public when I was signing people up for the race at Asda. A woman told me she was disgusted that the run was taking place outside her house. I explained that it had benefited five charities, but all she said was, 'Why can't you go and run in another park?' That was such a successful run that I would like to know if she still feels the same. I understand that it can cause an inconvenience but it is only for a couple of hours on a Sunday morning and it really does help so many, not only through the financial gain for the charities involved but also through making the people of St Helens more active.

In that first year my target time went out of the window because I was pulled out doing other things on the morning of the run. At 6am I was putting banners up, I had no breakfast apart from half a bottle of Lucozade before the race began rendering all the training I had done beforehand pointless. The event worked, 700 people signed up for it and it was great to see people lining the streets to cheer on the runners. It took me 55 minutes to complete the course, which was pleasing given my poor preparation. Royce Simmons, Saints' coach at the time, ran it as did the club's conditioner Matt

Daniels, who finished in 12th. Former Wigan and Great Britain loose-forward Phil Clarke was the big surprise – he came in at 18th and my wife Linzi did it in just over an hour in the first year.

For the second race we stumped up £14,000 in advance to stage it and close the road, which is a big outlay, but we took the entrance money and tried to interest sponsors. However, it would have been our necks on the line if the numbers had fallen short. That said, 1,300 people registered and it was another big success. For the second race we finished at Saints' big new stadium. Langtree Park added something special, giving us a landmark place to finish and Saints were great with us in allowing us to use the facilities. Saints opened the North stand to runners' families allowing 2,500 spectators to watch the finish, making it special for every runner.

Saints' chairman Eamonn McManus and CEO Mike Rush have been very supportive of the Foundation, especially on occasions like this where the club and the ground staff have been co-operative in helping as much as possible. Eamonn presented the trophies and medals at the second race but probably didn't expect to be shaking hands with over 1,000 people but he did it for us and that was fantastic.

In the build up to the second race we did a few publicity stunts to grab a bit of media attention, and I did key parts of the course dressed in the costume of Boots, the Saints mascot. You'd think this would be a doddle and I figured I could keep taking the head off if I needed a breather. However, I had not banked on there being so many kids about, and given the furry mascot is as real to them as Father Christmas, I had to play the part of Boots, high-fiving dozens of children en route and bizarrely even having grown-ups coming up giving me hugs. I had to be Boots for the day and we had video of it all along the course which was a gimmick that really worked.

As for my own involvement, after the second race I was doing the Paris and London marathon challenge not long afterwards, so I had to be cautious. Unfortunately, I pulled my calf shortly beforehand and my physio advised me not to run the 10K course at all. That was not an option for me so I lightly jogged it with Mike Denning. Linzi beat me on this occasion but I enjoyed the run. It was better for me because I was able to talk to the people who wanted to speak to me. You can't do that when you are running full out – I enjoyed the interaction and that was good for me. I still had to be there at 5.30am to set up the banners and railings.

We keep increasing our numbers each year and have grown from 700 participants in the first year to more than 1,800 for the third race. It is nice in the build up to see people running in the streets and wonder if they are training for the 10K and in all reality they probably are. There were so many people tweeting and talking about the third race that I couldn't believe how many people were trying to get fit in St Helens. It was fantastic – that was one of the aims, to get people active.

Everybody knows that running is hard but you just have to be mentally strong to get people through it. Through keeping fit and active, it meant I was healthier and could cope with things like chemo, operations and rehabilitation better.

If the 10K was an activity, the idea behind launching the Pride of St Helens Award was to do something to celebrate my town's achievements in the world of sport, entertainment and industry. Despite any problems the town has, we are still prolific at producing real stars in a wide range of fields. As a town we are not very good at blowing our own trumpet and yet there are a lot of positive things happening in St Helens. That is the main objective of the Pride of St Helens – we need to let everyone know what is good about this town. The first ceremony was hosted in autumn 2012 and because we had never done it before there were some difficulties.

Pride of St Helens was mine and Martin's idea. We work quite well together and Martin takes over the organisation. We cannot do it without the help of people in St Helens. The sponsors are great and the *St Helens Star* has been tremendous in publicising the event and gathering the nominees. The night at Langtreee Park was a huge success and there were some fantastic awards and some great guests – actress Carley Stenson, world title contender Martin Murray and inaugural winner Andy Reid. To show the abundance of riches we had, Carley beat Johnny Vegas for the entertainment award and Martin Murray topped the sport category. As for the event itself, I would like to think it will grow, with more people doing good, positive things.

One of the other parts of the brief the Foundation has set itself was to put on fun, sporty events like the one we have staged at Taylor Park for some years now. We are using a big park that doesn't get utilised much, and the rangers have been supportive. Over the years we have staged lots of events – archery, segway, orienteering, running, It's a Knockout and using the big lake for dragon boating. It started off as a fitness challenge but now it has evolved into more like a day of sporty fun.

22

Disciplinary

One morning I received a call from Steve McNamara, who told me that the RFL were looking for people with experience to sit on the Match Review Panel. The panel is made up of people who scrutinise all the weekend's matches looking for illegal play before referring their findings to the Disciplinary Panel. He gave me the option of the disciplinary itself or the review panel and so I opted for the latter after speaking to, and taking advice from, the then England coach Tony Smith. After an interview with RFL, they offered me the job and seemed glad to get me on board. I could see why, because when I first went there were a lot of ex referees like Steve Presley, Neil Shuttleworth, Gerry Kershaw and Ian McGregor but no past players. It was my first job after coaching, playing and teaching. It took me three hours to analyse each game and then write all findings and present them to the other panel members. Every weekend we were given an allocation of Super League games to watch – and we would be given discs with a brief to watch every single tackle. The review panel makes a decision and then the disciplinary takes it forward to prosecute.

On my first day I thought to myself, 'Hold back and watch', but I opened my mouth straight away and was quite forthright with my opinions. I did not particularly want to do that at this early stage – but I enjoyed it all the same. The panel tries to be consistent, but in 2011 coaches called asking why some incidents hadn't been referred or complaining that others had. It is not the best process but they were always looking for ways to improve the process and we were good at listening. Part of me was nervous about being involved in making a decision that was going to see a player banned and lose money, but at the end of the day it was about improving the game, and watching out for the players' safety.

It was a pretty basic operation and you would not believe the room and equipment we were given. It was essentially a broom cupboard at Carnegie College. There were refs shirts hung up all around, a cheap telly and generally quite shocking resources. The team has subsequently moved to the RFL headquarters at Red Hall. Hopefully, the resources have improved also.

The tackle is one of the biggest things that has changed over the years since I stopped playing. It is now wrestling and grappling techniques that have come into play. There are lots of underhand moves including chicken wing, cannon ball and ninja – and it is the job of the panel to pick them all up. As a panel member, you are under pressure to make sure nothing is missed and you need to keep up to date with techniques. Taking action against the ninja, which is applying force through the knee, stemmed from Saints' Samoan prop Maurie Fa'asavalu needing a knee reconstruction after falling victim to it. One season we had three or four such knee reconstructions. Some of it is accidental but for some we watched the same players using the same technique every week.

The chicken wing, which is pulling the arm back to put pressure on the shoulder joint, came over from Australia. We have watched some clubs develop this even more and hold the tackle while the third man comes in. Sometimes the timings are wrong but it is difficult to punish some players because of the way the law was phrased. The laws need to change but cannot change half way through a season, which is frustrating.

There were things we identified where no action was subsequently taken. On one occasion we sent up an incidence of roller pin, which is kneeing or dropping on the back of someone's leg. The response from the disciplinary was, 'Don't send any more of these up, there is nothing wrong with them.' We, on the Match Review Panel, could see players slowing the play the ball down by kneeing, it was a tactic that could cause injury on the back of the knee and leg, but they said they had no issue with them.

Fans have a real perception of inconsistency but you have to take into account the rules. The cannonball tackle caused a furore when the attack on the leg of Warrington's David Solomona in the Wigan cup tie went unpunished because it was not deemed a standing leg and the player was still moving. It badly hurt the player but could not be judged an illegal tackle – the law has since been changed.

In my last year on the Match Review Panel, 2011, I felt we had some poor calls from the disciplinary committee. The match review and disciplinary panel are two separate bodies and it was sometimes frustrating for us. For example when Ryan Bailey was sent off we sent it up and the three people on the disciplinary panel said 'guilty' and banned him. He appealed it and then two different people overturned it and he was off the hook. It's not right that two people can overrule what had already been decided and that is why fans can see inconsistency.

I hope it benefited the disciplinary process to have an ex-player on board – but after a few years it's easy to fall into the system and so you need a new person to come in to make you think. In 2011 they brought a coach on board in Jon Sharp, and he had a lot of new ideas, as did former Halifax forward Paul Dixon. The players in the collision are improving and developing their techniques all the time. They are all trying to get to the next level by adopting techniques to slow down the play the ball. Players when they are tackled now are probably thinking about the third man coming in from somewhere and concentrating on who is going to hit them.

At the meetings I asked how we could improve ourselves and requested being able to watch England wrestling or go into a club to see them train. The answer was no because clubs wouldn't want that in case they were doing something wrong, which is fair enough, but it was hard to understand why we couldn't use the England team because they are independent. It was hard to update our knowledge as a result.

There were times when I thought we were on a bit of a hiding to nothing and every Monday we expected a coach to phone. Tony Smith, when he was England coach, probably had a part to play in organising the structures this way. However, when he went to Warrington he was constantly ringing up to say he didn't agree with what we had done. On one occasion Tony blew up on Sky complaining about something we had done and that really annoyed everybody on the panel. There was a view that he was supportive of this idea when he was in charge of England, yet he washed hands of it when he became a club coach again. I suppose you change your views to suit your role.

Banning players is tough because they lose money, pay fines and miss games, but the panel has a job to do. I could explain things from a player's point of view outlining why they had done particular things. There were a few incidents where I knew players involved but I had to be professional. It was tougher towards the end, people started to become aware that I was on the Match Review Panel. It was hard because one week I would be involved in making decisions against somebody, yet the next week I may be asking the same player if he wanted to get involved in a charity event for the Foundation. I consciously did not make it known publicly that I was on the panel because of all the negativity about the whole process of banning and not banning players. I remember one week we were told that Sky's *Boots n All* wanted to come in to do a piece on the role of the Match Review Panel. As a joke I turned up for work wearing a balaclava, laughingly telling them I wanted to remain anonymous, not only for the reason above but also because I didn't want people to know I worked in a broom cupboard. The panel are there to help protect players but that is almost put to the bottom of list when there is an outcry over someone missing a big game through suspension. Hopefully, the stigma will change within the rugby league community. Overall, it was a good experience and I enjoyed the people I met there and had some good laughs on the way. You can't do anything but laugh when you are working with Steve Presley. I made some really good friends, even if it did mean working all weekend and having early starts on a Monday morning. Best of luck to all the panel members!

23

Return to Coaching

It really does not seem that long ago since Saints 'A' team coach Frankie Barrow was pushing skinny old me through the ranks and helping me to get a full-time contract. Returning to St Helens at the start of 2012 saw me turn full circle and I was the one giving coaching and guidance to young players to help them get a break.

The job assisting the coaching staff at Saints under 20s and 18s allowed me to be involved in my hometown club again 15 years after reluctantly departing as a player. An advert for community development workers at the club triggered my thoughts that it was time I got full-time employment. There were questions in my mind, like can I handle the workload and would it work with me still needing scans, my Foundation work and balancing that with my family life and spending time with my children. I was also concerned about the impact that siding with one team again could have on the Foundation. I only had a few days to get my curriculum vitae together, something I had not done for quite a few years.

I then got a call from Mike Rush, the now CEO at Saints. He asked me to get involved with the under 20s in a part-time role working with Glyn Walsh under Ian Talbot. I also spoke to Royce Simmons, who was first team coach at the time, and I found some common ground with him. The straight-talking but likeable former Australian Test hooker had attended the boxing event we had staged in Sutton when he first took over at Saints. He was also a bit of a runner, too, who once did five marathons when he was coach at Hull in the early nineties in order to raise funds to sign

Australian half back Des Hasler.

I already had close links with Saints anyway and those were cemented further when Royce asked Andy Reid and me to speak to players in a classroom ahead of the 2011 play-offs with the brief 'to try and be inspirational'. It was a difficult thing to do and I was quite nervous because I knew a lot of the players, but I think I did fine considering it was off the cuff. Andy spoke about his time in the army in Afghanistan before he was blown up by an IED that cost him three limbs.

It was hard going back into professional sport, but the lads were good to me and showed me some respect. My job with the under 20s was about helping those lads get a step up into the first team. It is simple, the good kids – that is the ones with potential to be Super League players – have got to start standing out and stepping up to the plate. I look back to when I was their age and I ask myself 'did I stand out when I was in the Academy?' Probably not! It is difficult because there are a of lot kids coming through and if you don't stand out at 20s you are not going to make it at Super League level. You have to be aware that some kids are not physically developed at that age. A lot are similar to me when I was their age and I only gained my physique and strength by being in the first team and doing weights. So I have to be careful not to be too critical of the young lads.

Coming back to the game worried me because I thought about the knowledge I had left behind since I had been forced to retire as a player. The game moves on and I thought it may have moved on too much – but it was comforting to find that rugby league is still essentially the same and I enjoyed working on the micro skills with the players, the passing and gripping the ball. So I was probably worrying for nothing, although I would have liked to get more knowledge about being an assistant. I felt I needed to be involved a bit more and so watched a lot of first team drills to pass that on to the 20s. My old friend Steve McNamara even allowed me to have a look at the England drills before the 2011 Four Nations. Maybe it is the lecturer in me, but I like to be prepared because I am frightened of failing or cocking things up. When I attended my first training session, I thought I had better not to tread on anybody's toes, but then I couldn't help myself from being forthright. Personally, I thought I was probably a little too bullish at first but if I was I can only apologise as the excitement of being back involved got the better of me. Mike Rush encouraged me to be open, as did my colleagues Ian and Glyn.

The big changes since my last game at Saints in 1997 were the facilities and the way a player's performance is analysed. It is a different world – with computers widely used to pick up faults and weakness, a fully equipped gym and a 3g pitch up at Cowley High School, as opposed to a muddy pitch in front of Knowsley Road illuminated by a few 50watt bulbs and some helpful car headlamps.

I was pleased with how the season went, as were all the coaching staff. We had built up good relationships and worked well as a team. There was no major pressure on us as coaching staff as it was about getting the youngsters developed and ready for first team and not all about results. We did however manage to finish third in the competition and completed an impressive home and away double over local derby rivals Wigan Warriors, then went into the play-offs needing to win against a strong Warrington team to make it to the final. Alas, we were beaten 42-22. On a positive note, 2013 saw some of these youngsters, step up and make the grade in the Saints first team: Nathan Ashe, Lewis Charnock, Joe Greenwood, Jordan Hand, Mark Percival, Dom Speakman, Adam Swift, James Tilley, Anthony Walker and Carl Forster.

Unfortunately, the Rugby Football League made a controversial decision to abolish the under 20s competition at the end of my first season. It was a shame as things were working; however after much deliberation it was decided that it would be replaced with dual registration, whereby Super League clubs can place their fringe players with partners in the Championships. Saints linked up with Rochdale Hornets, Ian Talbot retained the Head Coach status, Glyn Walsh and I teamed up with Matt Calland and Dave Ramsbottom, both existing Rochdale staff as his support. Would this work?

It could have been a recipe for disaster; you know the saying 'too many cooks spoil the broth'. Well on the contrary – it worked from the start. All the coaching staff gelled and it is so far so good. I already knew Matt from my playing days and Dave is a great bloke. It takes the pressure off, especially for me. If I am not feeling too great or if I am in hospital, I know the backup is there and I don't feel like I am letting them down so much.

The coaching style hasn't really changed but the personnel have.

Ian has been under pressure to recruit new players and to try to find that winning formula to help gain promotion. Rochdale are now a club with excellent facilities, a great foundation to build on, committed playing staff and great team spirit. Hornets had been a struggling club prior to adoption of the dual registration system. They were aware that changes had to be made, so this was a great move for them. The fact that they hadn't won many games meant that the players didn't have a 'song'. All clubs have a club song which is sung in the changing rooms after a win. One of the lads, laughing, said, 'Why would we have a song, we didn't need one last season – we never won!' That was going to change so they have now all learnt, 'Hornets we are ready, ready!' and it has been used on several occasions.

I am enjoying the challenge and working with everybody involved at Rochdale, from the back room staff right through to players and coaching colleagues. Hopefully Hornets will build on 2013's success and maybe, who knows, one day they will make Super League.

24

Recognition

Although I never got into charity work for awards and recognition, I have in fact been lucky enough to be invited to some prestigious events and fortunate enough to earn some highly regarded honours.

The first bit of recognition for my work for charity came from the RFL, when I was invited to kick off the All Golds game at Warrington. There was no big fuss, it was all a bit rushed really – I got changed in one of the offices in the reception area at the Halliwell Jones Stadium, ran straight out on to the pitch, kicked off, shook hands, got changed and took myself off home. Looking back it was a great honour and the kick off wasn't that bad mind, even though I wasn't at my strongest then. The Foundation was allowed to do a bucket collection that night and we made an amazing £3,000.

In 2009 I was awarded with the special honour of The Spirit of Rugby League award which is named after the late Mike Gregory. This was presented at the Man of Steel awards and was particularly special. It was supposed to be a secret, but ahead of it, Sky journalist Angela Powers came around and interviewed me for *Boots'n'All* and said they were doing a piece on me. It was a deep, thorough interview where they took me out around the park with my family. Two weeks after that bit of filming I lay in bed and thought why has that piece not been shown on TV yet? Although they were all trying to keep it a secret I started to think something was happening. I didn't prepare a speech for that night in case it was all in my mind. But I am usually good at reading situations and working things out. So an off the cuff acceptance speech was the way I went that night. Speaking is definitely not my forte but I am without doubt getting better the more I do. I suppose being unscripted works better sometimes if you know what you're talking about and people can tell you're sincere when you talk from the heart, so I think it went well. I had been coached by Mike at Saints when he was Shaun McRae's assistant so I knew him personally because he was one of my first coaches.

His wife Erica presented the award to me, but unfortunately I didn't get chance to say much about Mike. It was basically a question and answer type interview with Sky's Eddie Hemmings and he was asking me about the year's challenges and my illness. It meant I didn't get the opportunity to say how much I really respected Mike as a person and as a professional which still passes through my mind with disappointment now. Thanks Mike, God bless and RIP.

Also in November that year I was awarded the Arthur Brooks Memorial Trophy, the RL Writers Award for services to the game. Past winners have included players, coaches, administrators and pressmen and to be acknowledged by the rugby league writers and media correspondents, who have a great knowledge and appreciation of the game, made me feel humble. It showed that they had recognised my efforts and what I was doing for charity.

Rugby league players very rarely get a look in when it comes to the honours system – there have been quite a few MBEs and OBEs handed out to our code in recent years, but they still have a long way to go to be up there with rugby union. So I was pleased and honoured to be awarded an MBE for services to rugby league and charity. The RFL nominated me and a few months later the kids collected the official looking envelope from the postman and brought it upstairs to us. Linzi and I anxiously opened it with anticipation. We thought it was going to be a tax demand so it was a pleasant surprise. It stated that I should not tell anyone but of course, I had to tell a few people, close family, although I was mindful that if it came out it could be rescinded.

Apart from the personal pride, I took this as an honour for rugby league – a fantastic sport that does not get the recognition it deserves. Although I am not doing the charity work for awards, I accepted this one with open arms. The award is not just for me, but also for my family, friends and all the special people who have been involved with the Steve Prescott Foundation. It was also a really special award for the kids because I know I am not going to be here for all of their lives. So for them to be able to look back and say their father has been awarded an MBE for helping people out and doing things, well what more positive message can I leave as a role model for my children?

As for the investiture, I went down to receive my award from Prince Charles at Buckingham Palace the same weekend as my second marathon in spring 2010. It was all a bit daunting really as we followed the red carpet in. I had obviously seen Buckingham Palace prior to this day, on sightseeing visits to the capital, however walking through the guarded gates and through the entrance was special.

Linzi and I decided to take our two young boys along as, after much discussion and debate, we thought it was an opportunity they shouldn't miss. My wife still claims she was more deserving of the medal that day after she was separated from me from the moment we entered the palace. I was whisked off into a grand room whilst I was coached on how to address the Prince. We were given countless do's and dont's on how to approach and retreat. All the time I was worrying about what I would say to him and pondered what he could ask me. On the other hand, Linzi had to take the boys, aged eight and three at the time, and keep them silent for two whole hours whilst all recipients individually came up to receive their honour. This proved almost impossible as Koby kept shouting out that he was bored and wanted to go back to the hotel. Linzi was so stressed and embarrassed she actually had to put her hand over his mouth and gag him on several occasions. It must have been very boring for them sat through the awards for hundreds of people they didn't know, so much so that Koby, the boy that never sleeps, fell asleep! When I entered I scanned the room and spotted my family, I was gutted to see Koby snoozing. I really wanted him to remember this when he was old enough to understand, after all that was the reason we decided to take him. He was woken just before it was my turn.

I approached the Prince as I had been instructed, but once he began to ask me questions about St Helens, my injury and the charity work, I relaxed and completely forgot about the etiquette. I had been told that once the Prince held out his hand that was the cue for me to take my two backward steps and bow to his Highness without turning my back to him. Well that went out of the window, because I was·the one who offered him my hand, when I realised what I had done I became flustered and very nearly turned around to walk away. I quickly corrected myself and looked up at the Prince, who gave me a knowing smile that I had very nearly cocked up. I was tormented about this but had to laugh when I watched it back on the DVD.

Honours give you a good feeling, but nothing was more pleasing than being asked to present the Challenge Cup at Wembley in 2010. The Rugby Football League invited me to be guest of honour, although I did have to pay for everything myself except for my seat in the Royal Box. I'm not moaning, but would they have asked Prince Charles to pay for his own train, tube, taxi and hotel? It was great that they afforded me the honour and I will never forget it, but the RFL accountants must have been made up at getting me so cheap!

That in no way took the shine off what was a tremendously prestigious occasion that left me with plenty of good memories. It was a fantastic honour to be a part of and I loved every minute of it, starting with the walk down Wembley Way with all the fans. Although it was a privilege to go out and greet the players during the pre-match presentation, I was initially worried what they would be like with me. I shouldn't have worried – there was a huge amount of mutual respect there and I was given a hugely warm reception from both sets of players and fans alike. As I walked down the line I received hugs off players like Garreth Carvell, rather than the more formal handshake. I had played with a few of these guys and the Warrington club have been really good, both with me and the Steve Prescott Foundation. Several players from both clubs had given time up and helped the Foundation in one capacity or another and I had good relationships with them. Leeds skipper Kevin Sinfield is a top bloke as well as a first class footballer. Kevin was in the team for my last ever game – that ill-fated Lancashire v Yorkshire clash where I broke my knee cap.

The daft thing was, when it came to the moment of glory during the winner presentation, my whole reason for being there, I nearly forgot about the big, shiny silver thing with ribbons on in front of me. Adrian Morley grabbed me when I was giving him his medal and he was so emotionally charged that it put me off what I needed to do. Richard Lewis nudged me – and said urgently, 'The cup, the cup.' Of course! It was fantastic to see the emotion of the Warrington players when Morley raised it above his head.

I watched the game alongside the then Rugby League boss Richard Lewis in the Royal Box, and he is a really nice person, as is Nigel Wood. They made us feel very welcome and it was a special occasion. At a later date I sat with Nigel at the Man of Steel awards dinner where I can remember him trying to give me dietary advice. 'If it is green, eat it' was his rule – but I was sat there thinking, 'How can I take dietary advice from you?' The whole situation made me chuckle. For those who don't know, Nigel is quite a hefty man, but he is infectiously enthusiastic about his rugby and a nice fella to boot.

In 2011, I was presented with an Honorary Degree from the University of Hull, honoris causa. Being honoured in the city of Hull made me particularly proud because it had played such a huge part in my life. It is where my two boys were born and where I enjoyed and played rugby for so long. The ceremony took place at the City Hall, in the city centre, with the Business School graduates. I was fitted with an academic robe, cap and gown, but had to Google the protocol and how to doff my cap.

Also in 2011, much to the surprise of many of my friends, *The Independent on Sunday* announced their Top 100 Happy people in Britain. Patricia Roffey and Emily Dugan presented 100 people who make Britain a better and happier place to live and I made this select band of people. Well I think this was the one that got me the most stick. Even my wife questioned whether they had called this one right. I was pleased but also saw the funny side of the honour. I think if you were to ask Linzi or my friends they would probably liken me more to Mr Grumpy than Mr Happy. Can you imagine the ridicule I received?

More recently, the town of St Helens has recognised my efforts and my desire to inspire others. At the new stadium, Langtree Park, I was selected as one of the players to adorn the concourse in the shape of a mural. The striking player murals have enriched the stadium with a sense of the club's proud history and proven to be a fantastic feature on the concourse and maintain links with the history at Knowsley Road. I was honoured to be one of a select group of players who all seem to be legends of this great club.

Also regeneration bosses within the town of St Helens were successful with an application to St Helens Council for an art work bench at Sherdley Park, which included steel silhouettes of me, comedian Johnny Vegas and a glass blower. It is surreal for my children to go to the park and see their dad in a permanent fixture so let us hope it stays free from vandalism.

At first the primary purpose of doing my challenges and charity work was to give something back, to help others like people had helped me and also to raise funds to help the causes I was backing. It hadn't really clicked in my mind that I could actually do something as grand as inspiring other people. I am quite a modest person and when people started approaching me and saying, 'You are inspirational,' my first reaction was shake my head and deny that and think to myself I'm just being me. That was how it was for a few years until I slowly began to realise that I must be helping and inspiring people as well. People continue to send me so many nice letters, saying they are doing this event or that activity to raise money to help others, or things like, 'My dad has cancer and is using you as an example of mental strength and the ability to not give up and fight it all the way.'

Even people telling me things like they are losing weight or giving up smoking, because they have seen what I have done and can relate to how I've fought this disease for so many years feeds back into me in a positive way. Sometimes I feel this can be more rewarding than the financial donations the charity receives. Regarding recognition, I suppose the more we get, the more it raises the charity's profile and earns money to help more people. So please don't stop giving and get involved in any event you feel like you are able to.

25

Paris to London

Again, another chance conversation with Martin and a few months later I was climbing up on to Paul Sculthorpe's shoulders to have our pictures taken underneath the iconic Eiffel Tower and the latest madcap challenge was underway. The plan was to run both the Paris and London Marathons on consecutive Sundays and in the week in between, cycle north to Calais, kayak the English Channel and then get back on the bike to London. We had a week to cross the channel because we were tied by the dates of the Paris and London marathons, and we were also very reliant on the weather conditions.

When I asked Martin who would do the challenge with me there was only one name on his lips, 'Scully!' Martin asked him and he said, 'Yes, yes, yes, I'm in.' True to form, Martin started planning the event straight away and suddenly it was happening. Leading up to it I was a bit sceptical that Scully was too fit and competitive – the sort of attributes you associate with a back to back Man of Steel winner. Although I did a little bit of training on my own, taking advantage of the limited oxygen cycling chamber at Saints training ground, I purposely did not do much with Scully. This was partly because I knew that it would wreck my head and secondly, there was a concern that I would be holding him back. However, because I wouldn't go training with him he didn't do enough either. As a professional sportsman you don't want to be the weak link, the one holding the other back but on this occasion it would be just the two of us and not a large group as in previous challenges. I was concerned that my illness could affect my performance on this extreme endurance event. There was nobody to hide behind, I would have to keep up with the machine that is Paul Sculthorpe or frustrate him by holding him back. That was just one of the worrying things floating around my head. In the end it was great having Scully there. He understood that it was not a competition between us, there were only two of us and the philosophy binding us was, 'Let's get to the end together.' The Tom Petty song 'I won't back down' will always remind me of that event. Scully and I listened to that song on numerous occasions and we have both grown to love it.

Before we set off we did have to do a bit of work on our kayaking skills and boy, what an eye-opener that was. Scully and I did five sessions out in rivers and lakes, including the River Dee. I fell in most of them, but the last one was the most testing and it was Scully who went in the drink. Our plan was to kayak the English Channel so to prepare ourselves for that we went out in the Irish Sea to Anglesey. We were in the bay initially and I thought that was bad enough but when we went out to sea we didn't know what had hit us. It was rough out there with a strong wind. We were complete novices at this game – Scully had gone quiet. My way of dealing with that was to burst out laughing but I did begin thinking, 'What the hell am I doing here?' It was so hard because you are on your own in the kayak – and I recall the instructor who was with Scully asking, 'Are you all right?' Next minute he had capsized, which was frightening at first because it seemed that he could not get out of his boat.

We had practised unlocking the spray deck and getting out of the boat at Sutton Leisure Centre, but it was a different ball game doing it in freezing cold sea water. I remember thinking that Scully was not coming out, then he bobbed up and went back under so I panicked a bit. He was frozen to the bone and then he went in again and I think that this experience showed a different side to Scully. Alan Pinnington, who took us out to sea, clocked what was happening and towed us to the port while Scully got himself together, but all I was thinking was that we have got to go back across these waters to get to our base. Kayaking, especially in such rough seas, means that your body's core is constantly working. Although I managed to get back to base, Scully was towed back and was freezing. This particular escapade was a week or two before we set off for Paris and it was a massive dent to our confidence. We now knew how hard kayaking was and how tough it was going to be doing this from Dover to Calais. On the way home in the car, it was the first and only time I have witnessed Scully questioning his mental strength ... but it didn't last long! When he got out of the car he turned to me and said, 'We'll smash it!'

The Paris Marathon was a great experience. We had some good laughs in the lead up. We had to travel over to Paris the day before, the registration in a foreign country added to the adventure. We had both been kitted out with sponsored clothing from Asics and we had to laugh when I announced that we looked like twins, me being Danny Devito and Paul, Arnold Schwarzenegger. Paris was Scully's first ever marathon. The furthest he had ever run before that day in training was 10 miles. Anybody else attempting a marathon after such little preparation would most certainly fail, however something told me that Scully would breeze it – and he did. On the day I kept telling him to go for it and leave me, after all this was his opportunity to set his personal best before the enduring days of cycling began the following day. Scully being Scully stayed with me to make sure I got through it. That's the kind of guy he is. He never once made me feel like I was holding him back, not just in the first marathon but during the whole event.

Scully stuck with me when I was starting to tire and get cramp, just as I had in my previous marathons, he was insistent and I kept thinking, 'crack on mate'. In the end I forced him to kick on with six miles to go and Scully ran his first marathon in 4 hours 22 minutes – he was so strong at Paris, especially considering the furthest he had run previously was the Great North Run half marathon. To run 26 miles with no problem was amazing. The last six miles were horrendous for me. The difficulty I found was that I had not done a marathon for two years and I'd forgotten how hard they are. Through my illness and the condition my body is in I have come to the conclusion I cannot run any faster. The fluids just go straight through my body so I have nothing left to give.

I let Scully go and struggled all the way home then. There were demons everywhere in my mind, but I had to battle through, and was grabbing French sweets and pretzels from people on the sidelines. The oranges they offered me were the nicest, most refreshing things I had ever tasted. That said, I was simply sucking the juice because my condition means that I can't eat fruit. My left calf and then my right hamstring cramped up but everyone was running past tapping me, saying, 'Come on!' which helped me over the finish line. Scully, who had finished three minutes before me, was waiting at the finish line. We went up for our medals but my legs had gone and my quads were not working. Thankfully we had taken a physio with us so could get a massage off Paul Head, but I was physically gone and worried how I would get up the next morning. There were no celebrations at the finish line, I was too shattered for any of that and had to prepare for the next morning. I knew I was in trouble. There was no rest day and we cracked on with the challenge by cycling 170 miles in two days straight after the marathon. It soon became clear that I had underestimated and underprepared for a challenge yet again. Scully and I laughed that we had winged it because the only time we had cycled together was a 15 miler around St Helens. There was no power in my legs and I struggle on hills at the best of times but it seemed every time we had a climb Scully was at the top, dismounted and waiting for me. That is the way it was and Scully accepted that.

After my cycling difficulties during the LEJOG challenge I made sure I was measured up for this one by Thatto Heath Cycles. My knees had caused a lot of problems so I made sure I got them right beforehand and was assisted by a very good physio in Lorna Wellens, who got the tracking right on my knee. Ever since I had broken my knee cap it has been tilted and wouldn't track right but we used the coloured tape that the athletes use to keep it in place.

The second day of the challenge was the worst day for me. It was a case of getting straight on the bike after the marathon to clock 110 miles from Paris to Abbeville. I could not walk, my legs were not working, and despite having physio, getting into an ice bath, wearing compression tights during the night, I was still stiff and sore the next day. It must have been bad because I couldn't get up or down the stairs at the hotel.

Running the marathon had taken so much out of me that with 30 miles to go in the bike ride I had nothing left. I badly needed some sugar, and had a can of coke and some Jaffa cakes and somehow got to the finish. I was gone – and was so completely fatigued that I felt like crying. Afterwards I was sat in the hotel reception and couldn't move for an hour.

On the third day we did 78 miles and then took the ferry to Dover. It was an awful day, the weather was bad, Scully got a puncture and while we were trying to mend it we could barely feel our hands. It was another day of massive hills but we cycled into Calais together.

Fulfilling the next leg of the challenge was even trickier. We had a two day window of opportunity to kayak the Channel. We had to come up with a plan B, if we couldn't cross on those days we would use the time to cycle from Dover to London to get that out of the way. However we were so exhausted that we took the Wednesday off. We went to see the sea captain that afternoon and sat around a table. The captain – Michael Orum – talked about the weather conditions. Shaking his head he said, 'Not looking good'. Straight away he said there was no chance of kayaking across the English Channel. He explained that all those wishing to kayak the previous week had not been allowed to because the weather was so bad. However, he showed us a five-man boat and gave us that option. It was the same type of boat that John Bishop had used to row the Channel for Sport Relief not long before.

Scully and myself are not the sort of people who shy away from a challenge, but when the sea captain would not let us kayak the Channel the feelings of disappointment were mixed with a massive relief. I assume Scully felt the same because his confidence had been knocked so badly by his dip in the Irish Sea during training.

We could not have pulled out – but when they gave us the 'five men in a boat' option we said, 'Yes, definitely.' However, even with that there were weather problems and we had little chance for the Friday but there was a possibility of crossing on Saturday. The captain showed us the model boat on his mantelpiece to explain what type of vessel it was. We were up for it although we did then have to convince him that we were quick learners and to take us across. We had done no actual rowing at all – just a lot of dragon boating which is paddling and not the same thing. We were also in the lap of the gods when it came to the weather.

After taking the Wednesday off we cycled to London the following day to get that bit chalked off. We got off to a flyer and even after being soaked as we got to London we were relieved that the cycling was now over. The bikes were in the van and not coming out again.

We then had the task of enlisting our crew for the channel crossing which was problematic because we had no fixed day or time. Although we had taken the initiative and started recruited people for the Friday, including *Emmerdale's* Kelvin Fletcher and former Great Britain and Wigan full back Steve Hampson, they couldn't make it on Saturday – so we needed a contingency plan for our contingency plan, so to speak. But that was the least of my worries. In the car on the way home from London I started to get the stomach pains that usually end up with me going to hospital – but didn't tell anybody apart from my wife. After all the work we had done I was mortified that this would be challenge over. My thoughts kept going back to the Keep on Running Challenge when I suffered from a bowel obstruction and I can usually tell when one is coming on. I thought this would be one of those occasions. Thankfully, it cleared up overnight without medical intervention.

Some of the people down in Dover must have thought me and Scully were nuts because every morning we walked into the stone cold sea. It was our way of just taking a natural ice bath. As we watched the sea and the weather, with time running out, former Saints captain Chris Joynt and former team-mate Bernard Dwyer both signed up, with Steve Hall making up the trio on standby up in the north. Bernard, who had no experience whatsoever of rowing, told us it was his 45th birthday on the Friday but count him in regardless.

We were told no chance for Friday so Saturday, the day before the London Marathon, was our very last opportunity. Martin Blondel pleaded with the sea captain to get us out, explaining how important it all was. The call came back that there was a window at 5am Saturday, so it was all systems go and the three lads headed south including birthday boy Bernard. He and Joynty had a few beers in the hotel on arrival but we had to get up at 4.30am to be at the dock for 5am.

The next morning we arrived at the docks to find that another group from Oxford University would also be making the attempt that day. After a friendly chat, reality soon set in when they informed us that they had been training for a full year and we had to laugh at their astonished faces when we told them that we'd had 24 hours notice. Unbelievably none of us had ever been in one of the boats we were about to cross the English Channel in. But they soon laughed back at us when they had asked about sea sickness and sickness tablets; all we had with us was packets of jelly babies and cereal bars. We then had to show our inexperience and ask the sea captain if he had any sea sickness tablets for us. Thankfully the sea captain came back with five – one for each of us.

Bernard then quickly went to the loo, mistakenly on their boat, and in true Thatto Heath fashion left a nice present for the posh boys. It was almost comical what we were doing – five Lancashire rugby lads, with no experience or training were about to row the English Channel.

We clambered into our boat and sat down making our first mistakes, we were facing the wrong way and Joynty was holding his oar upside down. The biggest laugh of the moment came when our inexperience really stood out as the sea captain informed us we would only be going around in circles as all five of us grabbed an oar. We stupidly hadn't twigged that we needed a cox. In fits of laughter we were pushed off, they didn't seem to see the funny side and I'm sure they must have had doubts on whether to allow us to make an attempt. We thought we would be quick learners but we crashed into the first boat before leaving the marina which we found even more hilarious. The sea captain and the other crew must have been thinking that these guys have no chance and, to be honest, upon leaving the marina so did we.

But we soon got the hang of it, turned it around and worked it out for ourselves. Although we tried to get in sync – with Hally as cox, me and Scully on the right and Joynty and Bernard on the left, once we hit the big waves and the swell it was frightening, so much so that we didn't look at the waves that were coming. The scary thing was that it was gale force four out there and we knew that our boat could not withstand anything beyond that. The sea pilots got worried, particularly as Dover did not seem to be getting any further away. We just carried on rowing.

We had taken food to sustain us but it became scattered about the floor of the boat with the waves we faced. We could not get to it without leaving our oars unattended which was a problem as if one of us did this, the boat became unstable as the sea was so rough. It was a case of grabbing at the cereal bars with one hand, opening it with your mouth and throwing drinks around if you got the chance. The experience became really scary! It was not what any of us had expected at all. Half way over after dodging the huge tankers, currents and waves, the dark clouds descended on us and we all went quiet.

Chris Joynt was sick and although it was unfortunate for him it brought some light to our frightening situation and we all burst into fits of laughter. The funniest thing was he didn't break his stroke and kept rowing throughout. The support crew we had brought with us were all sick from really early on because the speedboat was just bobbing over the waves. They couldn't even look over at us never mind speak or encourage us. Linzi and Martin were on board the speedboat. They were supposed to be filming us and be there as back up, but for about three hours they were too ill to do anything. Every time I looked over at them, one of them was spewing over the side of their boat. At one stage their boat actually run into us and knocked Joynty off his seat. This was particularly annoying for us as it was the professional sea captain's job to make sure we were safe and it was them that put us in danger. We later learnt that it was at that time when they were particularly worried for us making it across that they momentarily took their eye off the situation because for a full hour of rowing in the open waters the boat never moved. There were some worrying times. It went dark for a spell, it was freezing cold and the rain came down. Linzi had shouted that we only had six miles to go, but when we asked an hour later we still had six miles left. We had literally rowed to a standstill and not gone anywhere. Throughout the journey we kept rowing as the big ferries and tankers passed us – thankfully they noticed us although we did get a bit of swell from them when they passed by.

As we homed in on Calais I had it in my head that we wanted to row all the way to the French coast, even though the sea captain kept barking at us that we had to stop 100 yards short. We turned a deaf ear to his orders and I said, 'Bollocks to it, we're going to hit the beach!' We kept rowing – because we saw the shore as the finishing line – but all the time the captain was roaring about it being £20,000 worth of boat, and giving us a bollocking. He was worried because we were right next to the port of Calais, where all the big ships and ferries were coming in and the swell was quite bad. Frustrating as it was, we did as he said and stopped short, rowing all that way without actually reaching land! It was only when we boarded the support boat to go all the way back that we actually realised how far we had rowed. It is classed as 21 miles but you row more because of the times you are rowing sideways as a result of the current. It took us seven-and-a-half hours rowing with another two-and-a-half hours for the journey back. The journey back was rough, so much so that Martin Blondel broke two vertebrae and was in serious pain, ending up in the care of Whiston Hospital on his return.

All in all it was a great achievement for the five of us – and well worth the anticipation and stress of the build up and the thoughts and doubts of not being able to complete. Afterwards Bernard said, 'Thanks for the opportunity.' And he meant it. He had given up his birthday celebrations with his family and he was thanking me! Bernard had given himself the smallest, scruffiest, old pad to sit on in the boat. He kept sliding off his seat when he was rowing. It had eye-watering consequences and the following day – the morning of the marathon – he sent me a good luck message by text. It read, 'If you want any motivation look at this picture of my arse!' There was a massive blister across his backside where it had rubbed and chaffed on the crossing. Another memory which still makes me giggle. Sorry Bernard!

It was just really good fun and it is still hard to believe that a group of rugby lads from the north, who had no coaching or experience of rowing and who had never even seen the boat, rocked up in Dover and rowed the English Channel in seven-and-a-half hours. We cracked it, it wasn't a record but it was a great achievement for such an inexperienced group. Without the three boys who stood in and helped us at such short notice, this leg of the challenge would have failed. I can't thank them enough as I have to say it is up there with one of the best and most memorable things I have done. It was something I had on my wish list and still can't believe we did it.

I was tired afterwards though and ate my food in the hotel reception – we had to head off from Dover to London almost immediately. I drifted off to sleep whilst waiting for my curry and the waiter woke me up. The floor seemed to be moving. I felt a constant weird, rocking sensation and I did not get rid of that all night. When we arrived in London, some of our friends, Steve and Katheryn White along with Lindsay Sculthorpe were waiting to welcome us. They had come down to cheer us on the following day and laughed at me rocking with the waves, yet on dry land in the hotel lobby.

Mindful that this was the eve of the London Marathon the physio Paul gave my calves a good rub. And then it was a quick bite to eat and off to bed.

The finale, the last leg of this extreme challenge, was going to be a big day. All the way through the experience Twitter had come into its own in building support and we made newspapers and television. We were told we were going to get a BBC slot with Sue Barker before the marathon. Our interview was scheduled for 8.37am at our start point at Greenwich – we had planned the timing to perfection until we discovered Cannon Street station was closed and meant we ended up running two miles, uphill, to get to our interview before the marathon. We were both sweating cobs and absolutely knackered – I had to answer a call from the producer asking where we were whilst I was running in desperation not to miss this prime time slot to raise awareness of the charity. They were great though and we went straight onto live television without time to prepare (apart from me telling Scully to mop his brow). Both Scully and I spoke and we managed to get our message across as best we could under the circumstances.

Physio Paul Head strapped up both my knees – and after a quick toilet stop we were all set for the marathon. There were a few celebrities in the VIP tent and we had our photos taken with Gordon Ramsay. He didn't have a clue who we were, and why would he? He was a genuinely nice bloke. He wished us luck but said he wasn't looking forward to it, so we told him what we had done in the build up and he thought that it was amazing. We were off; the last leg of the most gruelling and intense week of challenges to date. Within the first mile Scully started struggling saying his 'glutes were really sore'. I told him to stretch – so he jumped into somebody's front garden, so not to get in anybody's way as the roads were crammed with people, and he did just that. We clocked the first mile in a time of 8minutes 37 and that includes stopping for Scully's stretching. Every mile we were ticking off at decent time and we fuelled early, got plenty of stuff in our bodies early. My goal, or maybe a tactic to gee me up, was to get to the half marathon stage with the logic being I could tell myself I have only got two hours to go. We got to that stage in 2 hours 5, so immediately the focus was to get to the 20 mile mark. At the 21 mile stage I got a bit of a twinge with cramp and Scully started struggling with his knee. For me it was a case of stop, stretch, walk, stop stretch, walk and then I could start running again – that got rid of it, but grabbing loads of sweets to get sugar in me helped too.

Scully, on the other hand, was struggling with his knee. He was clearly in agony with it and he was getting slower and slower. I kept trying to encourage him over last five miles. It is not hard to motivate someone like Scully – a fearless, skilful athlete who has won everything in the game and even took it to the Aussies. Although he was limping I turned to him and said: 'You are a double Man of Steel ... you have run through brick walls and smashed everyone in the game ... don't let this beat you, get yourself to that finish. Your job is to get me to that finish line.'

At 23 miles I looked at the clock and made a decision to go for it. I still had a chance of getting a PB and turned to Scully and said, 'I can get my PB here – are you coming with me?' He just nodded and said yes – what a transformation. We picked the pace up so much, when everyone else around us was wilting, that we were weaving through so many slow, struggling, broken bodies that were now littering the course. It was an amazing sight – we were literally pushing people out of the way to get past. I looked at Scully at the side of me and we were going full pelt and I thought, 'How are we doing this? Where has this come from?' It was hard to believe that suddenly Scully's limp was gone and he was flying. This just shows what mental strength can do.

The last three miles seemed to last ages but we kept going and going. I don't know where the energy came from, but I do believe Scully's winning mentality – drawn from years of winning Challenge Cups and Super League titles with Saints and scoring tries to win Ashes Test matches against Australia – was transferred to me for those last three miles. I had gone from thinking, 'I am injured and knackered' to 'I am going to kill it'. It definitely bounced back to me and helped me and was so good to see.

We got through a quite agonising last 800 metres around Buckingham Palace and then Scully grabbed my hand and lifted it up. He wanted us to cross the line together. It was a great feeling and I was absolutely buzzing off it. When I looked up and the big clock was showing 4 hours 23 – my fastest marathon to date – I was so made up. My previous ones had been 4.32, 4.24, plus a 4.25 in Paris seven days previously. Setting a PB was amazing given what we had done in the week's build up. I was so delighted and thankful to Scully.

Straight after crossing the finishing line we were round to Sue Barker for another BBC live interview and I was very excited and you could see that in the broadcast. Having done what we had done the day before and then to find the energy and will to win in the last three miles was tremendous. It was amazing that we actually ran the last three miles quicker than the opening three. I told Sue Barker, 'If you want to run a PB, row the English Channel the day before.' Sue did get a bit flustered interviewing us – at one stage she said we had rowed the Atlantic and I smirked a bit. Now there's a thought for the next one.

Of all my challenges to date, this was the biggest achievement – and I can't believe what we did on those last two days. Scully and I had made a good team and later he admitted that the best thing he could have heard in those crucial last few miles was my instruction that his job was to get me across the finish line. It focused him to do what he has always done in his career. Although he had his career cut short with injury, you can see there is still that strong competitor burning inside him. He had already shown that for the Foundation when he got into the boxing ring with heavyweight Brian McDermott. I got to know Scully well on the trip. He is such a great lad and good friend now and it was good having him along. In fact I needed him to pull me through on this one so I am so glad we asked him and he agreed.

I hope he can do more. Having done marathons in two capital cities, I feel the London Marathon is far better than the Paris Marathon. There are more characters, with more folk in fancy dress and it is really well organised, particularly at the start. It added to the atmosphere meaning it was not demoralising to be beaten over the finishing line by someone dressed as Tom the Mole.

Although I was quite sore afterwards, thankfully we both got a massage in the VIP area, something we have never had before. Athlete Ewan Thomas spoke with us and Scully explained the Steve Prescott Foundation's work to Gordon Ramsay, whose wife offered to make Scully a cup of tea.

Physically it took me three days to get over the challenge, but mentally it was a different matter. I was back in the gym three days later and people said I must be mad. It had to be done because I was on such a high and was even googling new challenges on the internet. But then bang, all of a sudden it hit me and I dropped. For two weeks I suffered, and was moody and not nice to be around. This is something that affected me before I finished playing rugby, after experiencing such emotional highs – I then faced a massive drop and was unable to cope with it.

Between us we raised over £22,000 for this event due to people's generosity. All credit to them for putting their hands in their pockets but it is small beer compared to the millions other sports stars like Ian Botham, Lawrence Dallaglio and John Bishop bring in through their challenges. Former England rugby union captain Dallaglio and cricketer Freddie Flintoff raised £2m cycling from Greece to London. That is what comes with being involved in a high profile sport. I don't get disheartened by that – the events we have done have been really difficult, especially for someone in my condition. At the end of day the Foundation can only do what it can do. If I can inspire someone to do something, then that is great because people can see what I am going through. We are doing the job and try to invent new challenges every year. One year I am certain someone will suggest going to the moon and back.

26

Race to the Grand Final: The 48 Hour Challenge

After the success of April's Paris-London double marathon challenge I felt as fit as I'd ever been and that gave me a great feeling. As such, adopting the adage that a challenge is not a challenge unless it is challenging, we decided to up the ante again in the autumn of 2012.

And so the plan for the Engage Mutual Race to the Grand Final 48 Hour Challenge was hatched. As is now the norm with these things the idea for the event came from Martin and I bouncing ideas off each other about what crazy things could we do next to capture the public's imagination. We explored different sporting fields and spoke about swimming the Humber and Mersey rivers in one day as a challenge. From there we expanded the idea, starting from a Humber crossing, working our way across the breadth of England from Hull to Liverpool by bike and, because rugby league is our heartland and background, we wanted to finish at Old Trafford and deliver the match ball to the 2012 Super League Grand Final. So we had to weave another couple of disciplines into that – adding running and canoeing to effectively turn it into a quadrathon. These were events that were going to test everyone and despite me being in the peak of fitness I can honestly say this was by far and away the most physically and mentally challenging event I have done. It was torture from start to finish.

We also made it hard on ourselves by compressing the event into 48 hours rather than spreading it over three or four days. Steve White, Martin and I discussed it first. Steve told us that it was achievable in that time span but we would have to cycle through the night to complete it. That aspect of trying to make the body perform in this extreme challenge without sleep was the difficulty that everybody faced. We had never done a challenge that involved sleep deprivation before.

It was made into a tough event because I wanted a test – and I was not alone, the other people who got involved with this also wanted to test themselves. You now see people who do Ironman challenges and triathlons – and there are plenty of people who want to train for something harder. A lot of people were involved and there were a lot of takers – 29 of us in total – despite it being a particularly tough challenge.

Ahead of the event my biggest worry was the swimming sections. I am not the strongest of swimmers, even though my ultimate goal at one time was to swim The Channel. However, after I had watched comedian David Walliams swim it and then after rowing across it myself I knew there was no chance I could ever do that. I approached my open water challenges with trepidation, starting off by getting advice and a wetsuit from Ribble Cycles, a company who have been great with the SPF and helped me out with different equipment. My training started straight away – building up the lengths in the nice warm pool at the DW Fitness is one thing, but swimming in open water is a different ball game. The water is so cold and I was a little frightened about what lurked underneath.

We did a bit of training at the Liverpool Docks but I ended up vomiting in the water during one of the training sessions because it tasted so disgusting. I kept thinking this isn't good for my health and my consultant had the same view and even suggested that I train using a snorkel so I didn't take much water in. There were even jellyfish in there and at certain times they seemed to be everywhere. So I decided to look for somewhere else to do my training. I ended up at Eccleston Delph, an old quarry site near Chorley where the water was much clearer. It was still cold and there were plenty of fish, including trout, in sight which unnerved me a little.

As for the logistics, Martin Blondel organised it all again. Although, we have our ups and down and argue about our opinions on which way the charity goes, we are like brothers really. Martin is paid, part-time, by the Foundation, so he has to make decisions on how to run the charity – but I have to have an input too because I want it to be right and it is my name being used. To our credit we have not failed a challenge yet. We have always come up with a plan B when things go wrong. And we did on this one – in fact we needed a plan C and D too. Unfortunately we persuaded Martin to delegate this one and put someone else in charge of sorting the Humber crossing, but late in the day we discovered that it had not been sorted out and that we could not swim the river. My biggest concern was how the rest of the group would take the news; after all we had advertised that we were swimming the Humber. It was all hands on deck and alternatives were sought. Richard Blowman, a local lad, organised for the swim to go ahead in a different location. However, the Humber Bridge was the iconic image so we decided to still incorporate it in the challenge. We started The Race to the Grand Final on the south side of the bridge and arranged a run across to where the bikes had been set up as Plan C was to cycle to Welton Waters where we swam the mile before we got back on our bikes. It was cold getting out of the water, but we had a hot meal, dried off and then got back on our bikes ready for a full night of cycling. It was not just the physical stuff, but I had a lot of talking to do to *Hull Daily Mail*, Sky, *Look North* and *Granada*. It is great coverage but it takes so much out of you emotionally. We cycled 50 miles or so to Wakefield before taking a break for soup and sandwiches. I was already pretty exhausted. Even though, as a player, I had not finished on a great note at Wakefield the club were superb with us that night and have been tremendous supporting us as a charity.

We had three cycling groups, with the stronger cyclists being done and dusted a lot quicker and were able to sleep while we were still going. They finished at about 3am, whereas we arrived in Liverpool nearer to 7am. The biggest difficulty was the weather and during the last stretch between midnight and 7am it was windy and pouring down. I was right at the back of the group, wobbling all over the road in the pitch black, struggling to keep up. As I was going over the Pennines I could just see, scattered in the distance, everyone else's brake lights. I was soaked to the bone and it was like a river coming off the hills at the side of the road. It was an awful experience.

We ate army ration packs on the planned stop to keep us going, not the nicest tasting things, but anything would have done because we were so hungry and tired. It was a really tough exercise and I could have quit so many times because I was so exhausted, but as always I was determined to get to the end. More often than not, I was at the front in my other challenges, apart from LEJOG which was cycling too. It took some of us 13 hours – with no sleep at all through the night – to get to Liverpool docks the following day.

When I got up, my body was a mess and I felt like I was jet-lagged, so I guzzled a can of Red Bull to try to get a lift ahead of the Mersey swim. We started off from the Wirral side of the river and swam towards Liverpool to the east of the docks area. Alas, there was again a glitch with the organisation and not enough support boats had been arranged. Waiting for boats, including some that never came, created a problem because we only had a certain timeslot before the Mersey current would change making it impossible to traverse. Basically the guy that was in charge of taking people across told us that there was not enough support boats. He put the fear of God into everyone when he gave a big talk to our gathering. He said, 'People can die here today.' He explained that not all of us would be able to go across and a lot of people in the group, once they heard words like dying, naturally took a step backwards. For some reason my mentality had changed. I had got myself back together; whether it was the Red Bull or simply my fighting spirit kicking in but I said, 'I am going over there!' Whether it was all the training I had done in preparation, or what I had endured the night before with the horrendous cycling stage, I was determined to cross the Mersey.

I declared out loud, 'I'm going over there, no matter what!' Sean Casey said to me afterwards, if I had not said that he would not have swam but after hearing me say those words he had to do it. I reckon even Scully had doubts but he had turned to me and asked, 'What do you think?' I replied, 'I am over there today.' Scully said he was in as well and stepped forward and was one of 11 out of the 29 that attempted the crossing. We had to come up with Plan E for the remaining 18 which was a mile swim in the docks – that disgusting water I had moaned about training in. All credit to them they did it, even Jimmy Gittins on his surf board, to complete the mile swim section on the banks of the Mersey.

But for those of us crossing the river, by the time we had waited for boats and listened to the bloke telling us about the risks and how unsafe the crossing was, I think we had missed the current time. It was going to be hard.

I had been practising with bubble wrap around me to help me float better, but I put too much on for this swim and looked like a Michelin man. With the River Mersey one side flows east and at the mid west it flows in the other direction. You have to swim accordingly to compensate. We swam in twos and I jumped in with Steve White, swimming with the current towards say Widnes-Runcorn way, and on reaching a buoy at half way point we would be heading towards the docks and the boats. I blocked out all the doubts and negatives as I front crawled across and was so determined that I did not even taste the foul water or feel the coldness. All I worried about was to keep my arms turning to get across. Looking up after half way, the bloke in the speed boat supervising us told me the tide was now really bad. He said that we would have to head back to the right and fight the current. Pointing out a red buoy about a mile away to our left he said, 'As soon as you are past that buoy you are out of the water and it is all over.' I did about 50 swimming strokes and looked up and the buoy went flying past me. I mistakenly thought the buoy was the one moving – but that was how fast the current was taking me. It took me a mile in 50 strokes. I powered as much as I could to get to the wall, which was 20 metres away but I was only about 20 or 30 metres from hitting the boats in the dock. I was yelling, 'It is there, the wall is there!' The man in the boat was yelling, 'Get out of the water ... now!' He went absolutely ballistic and roasted me, frightening me into getting out. I got in the boat and Scully and Steve White were already in there. He had picked most people up but I looked up and a few had made it out of the water and it was fantastic to see. I just wished one of them was me, but I gave it my best shot. I am not a strong swimmer and yet I was only 20 metres from the wall and I was made up that I had attempted it. I had mentally overcome some barriers, it had been so hard in the night and yet I attacked those doubts. I had no fear and wanted to do it. It was brilliant and I felt strong when I finished as adrenalin must have been flowing.

Triathletes Rob Hall and Dave Morgan managed to get across

and Howard Newall from The Christie also made it. The officials told me I had completed it, but I was disappointed that I had not got up the ramp.

There was no rest once we got out of the water – we changed at the boat house at Queens Dock and ran a half marathon to Runcorn Bridge that night. I knew that at the end of the run I could get a good night's sleep and a meal. I jogged, walked and ran but finishing the day was a big incentive. Everyone was tired due to the lack of sleep, so it was important to get a feed and a good night's sleep ahead of canoeing the next day.

Scully and I were in the canoe together when we set off at 6.30am. We had not trained, but had done lots of kayaking together in April. The Bridgewater Canal to Manchester is not violent water but it was all about timing with the other guy in the boat with me. I had never been in a two man team with Scully – but you realise how powerful a bloke he is and I had to compensate all the time. Scully was the power at the back paddling one side whilst I was at the front constantly fighting against Scully's strength for 27 miles. He was a great bloke to be in with.

The good thing about this last leg was that everyone was still with us – nobody had dropped out even though Jon Neill had struggled with his knee. Running is tough for a big bloke with knee trouble from rugby. Being cramped in a boat won't have helped him either.

It was hard. 27 miles is a long way when you are powering a boat yourself with no motor. We made this last leg light-hearted and more enjoyable than the previous legs by having a few stops at pubs along the way; this gave us the opportunity to meet some of the fans going to the game.

In one of the later stops it was suggested that Jimmy Gittins should get in our canoe so that he could take the ball over the finish line. The canoes were only two man but we kind of improvised and put him in the middle of us. Jimmy had done every leg of the challenge. He did the mile swim in Hull and Liverpool on a surf board. He was first in the water at Hull and wanted to do the challenge. It is fantastic that our charity can offer these chances to people with spinal injuries. Can you imagine how he must have felt after doing that? He was on the quad bike for the run and cycle legs and took part in whole event. It was so rewarding for me to see that.

However, in hindsight it wasn't safe really to put him in the boat with us and getting him in was difficult enough. I dread to think what would have happened if the boat had capsized because Jimmy was sat on his life jacket rather than wearing it – instead of sitting him on top of the bench he slid his legs underneath the bar for his comfort. We hadn't thought of the consequences or the health and safety of doing what we did but we just wanted him in the boat when we crossed the finishing line. We shouldn't have done it but it all worked out fine and nobody was hurt or injured. When all the boats were together with Old Trafford in the background, it was a great feeling. We made it and completed this extreme challenge with 15 minutes to spare.

At Old Trafford I did the coin toss with Leeds skipper Kevin Sinfield and Warrington counterpart Adrian Morley – and the fans there knew what we had all done in the build up. There was quite a theatrical show before kick off, with the ball being passed to me by an acrobat to put on the spot.

There were 29 of us that attempted and completed the event, but I am the figurehead of these challenges and as much as I don't want to take the entire spotlight when everyone has taken part that can happen. I have come to realise that in order for the charity to grow and gain awareness I have to take any publicity offered and if that means putting my face out there then it's something I have to do. I find it difficult as I feel like I am getting all the attention and praise like being down there on the pitch when the rest of the team, who have more often than not helped me get through, are sat in the stand watching me. I'm sure they must feel like they should be with me after doing the same challenge as me, but it is obviously not down to me or the Charity. That is the difficulty – but I hope they do understand.

Linzi and I watched a bit of the game but I was so tired that we went after half time – that was another big challenge completed. Who knows what that challenge took out of me? I don't regret doing it – training for it had kept the disease at bay and I think the consultants thought the same way as well, so I will never regret any of the challenges I have completed.

27

Only a Cure Will Help

Prior to the 48 Hour Challenge in October 2012 I was happy and would go as far as to say I probably felt the fittest I had been for a long time. How things change. Shortly after completing that event I started with excruciating abdominal pains and, believing I had another bowel obstruction, took myself to nearby Whiston Hospital. This had happened so frequently that I was well known to the A & E staff and also the SAU, but this time I couldn't pin point what I had eaten to cause the obstruction. This was unusual because I would always know. I would say 'this will be the tomatoes I ate at lunch time' or 'wild rice will be the cause of this'. We racked our brains but just couldn't think of anything. The hospital quickly told us that my electrolytes were low which would cause my system to slow down and effectively cause an obstruction to somebody with my condition, someone with an ileostomy. Around the same time the site around my stoma became sore and over a period of a few weeks a lump began to appear through the skin. In the first instance I thought it was a hernia perforated through the abdominal wall so made an appointment to get Dr Mark Saunders' opinion. After looking at it he didn't think it was hernia or bowel, but suggested it could be solid tumour that had made its way or been forced out. We were horrified and wondered what was going on inside and whether things were progressing. Linzi kept reassuring me saying, 'You were great three weeks ago; things can't have changed so drastically,' and reminding me that this disease is a slow growing tumour.

Dr Saunders arranged for us to speak to the surgeons at The Christie so they could have a look and give their advice on the matter. We waited a while, then we were shown to that very same room where we had been six years previous when we were told they couldn't do the 'big op'. We both felt eerie. When the surgeon came in his first words were, 'Here we are again, same room as six years ago, when we told you we couldn't do anything for you.' That wasn't the best start but it showed that my case had stuck in his mind, after all he must have seen hundreds of patients between those meetings.

He looked at the site in question and confirmed that it was a tumour making its way out. He went out of the room to take a look at my recent scans to see if this was a sign of progressive disease. We were both nervous and probably felt the same fears as we did six years ago. On re-entering the room he began, 'Well Mr Prescott, every time I look at your scans it amazes me how much disease you have in your body.' My heart sank. That wasn't what I wanted to hear because I knew I had widespread disease but didn't need reminding of that and switched off.

My mind was working overtime and I didn't want to listen to anything else he had to say. Linzi knows me too well and again she realised that he had knocked my confidence so she reinforced the fact that my scans had remained stable since my operation in Basingstoke. Linzi made him think a bit and then he actually admitted that he thought they were wrong at the time not to give me a chance and do the operation. It made me feel better that he had said that, but this encounter made me go away thinking, 'How long have I got left?' That was something I really hadn't asked myself for some time. In the car going home we both had tears and felt the weight of the world on our shoulders.

I am sure he didn't mean for us to react in such a way and he didn't realise that it knocked me back more than he will ever know but I was probably the lowest I had been for a long time. Linzi was upset, too, but she tried to remain strong for me saying, 'You're no worse off than you were before you went into that room. Nothing inside your body has changed – don't let him change what is in your mind, don't let him get to you.'

After a while I picked myself up. I had to; I wasn't going to get better moping around and realised once again that he wasn't the right surgeon for me and told Dr Saunders my concerns and, as always, he was great. He is such a people person, who knows how to communicate and has always been positive with me – that's what I need.

Dr Saunders suggested it was time for me to have another course of chemotherapy. The scans still showed stable disease but I had been treatment-free for four years and he felt it would be beneficial for me to be proactive rather than wait and have to be reactive. Deep down I knew it wouldn't be long before I needed chemo because I had begun to feel like the disease was creeping up on me. Even though I was worried and concerned about the side effects, especially over Christmas, I had been through it before and come out the other side. However, I had forgotten quite how bad the reactions were to the cold and was back to wearing gloves when going in the fridge and cold drinks were now out of the question.

The plan was to have another 12 cycles of the same chemotherapy as last time. It had helped to keep me stable and I tolerated it fairly well. There was talk at one point to opt for a different type, although they both had similar responses, the side effects differed. The options were going with the one which I had already had and knew how it would affect my body or the alternative that would mean I would not be affected by the cold but would more than likely make me lose my hair.

Letting Dr Saunders decide seemed the best option and he decided to stick with what I knew. He said both were just as effective but knowing how I liked to wax my hair and how I tolerated the oxaliplatin last time, it was a case of 'better the devil we know'.

I didn't really mind. I know needs must and I had to go with what was going to work best, but Linzi was relieved at his choice. Although Linzi would never have had any objection she didn't want me to lose my hair if there was an alternative. Her reasons were for our boys' sake. Although we were living with this nightmare, the hair loss would have made it real. She didn't want people to look at me and feel sorry for me because that's not the type of people we are.

The treatment started in November, funnily enough almost the exact time as the last session four years earlier. Learning from how I tolerated it back then helped Dr Saunders to plan for this time round. He made the decision to do it over two weekly cycles on a reduced rate to help lessen the side effects. The infusion was still over a two hour period, every other Thursday, however this time round we had the luxury of it being in the brand new, state of the art trials unit which had been built since my last lot of treatment. Alongside the infusion I also had to take the Capecitabine tablets for nine out of 14 days before the cycle would begin again.

In the beginning everything was fine, with the exception of the painful infusion which resulted in me having to put a heat pack over my arm to help reduce the pain and the random spasms in my hands and fingers, but overall the side effects were minimal. Linzi and I saw 'chemo day' as a good opportunity to sit down for three hours together and work on this book. It was hard to find quality time at home to do it with one thing and another in our busy lives. I started to look forward to it instead of dreading it like the previous times as I enjoyed reliving my life through the book.

However, as the cycles increased, the side effects increased too and it started to get harder for me. My body wasn't recovering as quickly between cycles and I began to lose weight. The numbness in my fingers became so bad that I struggled to button up my own shirt. So after nine out of the planned 12 cycles, Dr Saunders said enough is enough. He advised that I should take a break from the treatment to see if I could put some of the weight back on and we could review again in a couple of weeks. However, within that time I suffered another obstruction and very soon after I endured another one. It passed after a few days and I was more desperate than ever to get out of hospital and get home. The reason for my desperation was that the St Helens 10K run was due to take place only four days later. I knew in my own mind I wouldn't be able to compete in it but I did intend to complete it, even if it meant walking the route. I was discharged on the Wednesday before and although I was still weak I was confident I would be able to do it. That was until the early hours of the Sunday morning. I started getting the stomach pains again and the sickness followed. I spent the night on the en suite floor in pain. As the night passed and I could see the daylight through the window I began to realise that this may be the first time when I could not take part in one of the SPF events. I knew it would happen one day but I didn't think, or want, it to be so soon.

Linzi told me to go back to bed, to forget about the 10K and get myself right. It was hard for me to admit defeat and still at 6am I said I may still try to walk the course. How could I not do it? I would be letting so many people down. In the end, after listening to Linzi telling me how bad I looked and how people would understand, I compromised with her and finally came to the decision that I would turn up and cheer people on but not attempt to do it. I knew deep down that I wasn't well enough but it was so hard. All sorts of things were going through my head but the response I got from the competitors was immense and not one of them made me feel guilty that they were putting their bodies through it for my charity. I think they could see that my body was going through pain, but of a different kind. I must have looked awful that day because I certainly felt it. I tried to do my bit by being on the start and finish line and helping to clear up afterwards but I was gutted that I missed taking part in the event.

From that day on I didn't feel right. Although the stomach pains settled I knew I had to watch what I was eating. I spoke to Dr Saunders and he suggested that I move more towards a soft/liquid diet. I did and for a few weeks it got me by but I was beginning to get weaker and desperately needed a holiday to try to pick me up. The boys were off school and good friends of ours very kindly offered for us to use their house in Spain to get the break I needed. It was a much needed week in the sun, although I had to stay away from solid foods, which was very difficult when Linzi and the boys were having lovely meals in the restaurants and I had to stick to soups – if I ate anything at all. It was now getting to a point where I was frightened to eat as I didn't want to find myself in trouble. When I did have something, even liquids, my bowel started making strange, very loud noises. It was so loud that it resembled a blocked drain and kept both myself and Linzi awake. In fact we were worried in case it was also keeping the neighbours awake in the adjoining town house.

One day we were sat around the pool and made a list of everything I had eaten to try to piece together what was going on. We got the ipad out and Linzi trawled the internet even though it is not always a good idea to type symptoms into Google for fear of what might come up. Linzi did and she found lots of forums where people were experiencing similar symptoms to me and they had been diagnosed with small bowel bacterial overgrowth (SBBO).

The more we read up about it, the more we were convinced that was what I was suffering from. On our return, I rang Dr Saunders. I filled him in on what had been happening, the loud noises and what seemed like intolerance to dairy products. I told him about Linzi's research and although he wasn't convinced it was the problem he was willing to treat me for it on the off chance. I also cut out all dairy products from my, now already very limited, diet. It seemed to work. The noises stopped almost instantly and I began introducing foods back into my diet.

However, this was short lived and five days later I began to suffer with abdominal pain. It was another obstruction and I knew what I was in for. At first I sat it out at home, in agony but refusing to go into hospital. It was all too familiar for me so I decided to wait at home until it cleared itself. It was Thursday evening and I knew I was in for a long and painful night but I was sure it would be cleared by the morning; after all I hadn't eaten much. It got to Saturday and I was still in bed in tremendous pain. Linzi told me to go into hospital and get some proper pain relief. I know it is hard for her to see me that way and I know she wants to protect the kids from seeing their dad in pain, but I kept thinking it had to clear soon.

But it didn't and when it got to 7pm, I couldn't stand it any longer and gave in. I didn't want to admit that this disease was creeping up on me but deep down I knew these episodes were getting closer and closer together. Linzi arranged for the boys to go to their friend's house, but Taylor is getting older and wiser and he realises that this isn't the norm. He is beginning to understand that things are not right. He got upset that night and asked, 'Why does this keep happening?' It was the first time he had really questioned anything. Linzi explained in the best way she could whilst still trying to protect him. How much longer could we do that for? 'You know your dad has got problems with his bowel, this is just another hiccup,' she explained. She tried so hard to be calm and not break down but inside I know she was hurting and it was breaking her heart. Koby on the other hand is much younger and innocent. He was more than happy to pack his bag and saw it as a good opportunity to stay over at his best friend Harry's house. It was going to be Easter Sunday the following day so both boys chose an egg to take with them for the morning. At times like these we realise how much support we have from family and friends and we are so grateful. We are very lucky to have so much back-up and help.

As Linzi drove me to A & E, I began questioning what was happening to my body. It had held up so well but now I feared it was failing. We were both quiet in the car on the way there. I'm not sure if we both sensed that this time was different, but it was now three days into the obstruction and there were no signs of it clearing. I went through the whole rigmarole of questions, tests and so on and I was admitted on to ward 4C of Whiston Hospital where I was known to most of the nursing staff.

I was given morphine for the pain and was treated the same as always with a conservative approach. To be honest I think the consultant may have been frightened to treat me due to my complex underlying condition. So it was a case of sit and wait. Ten days passed, I had not eaten; I was deteriorating and could feel myself wasting away. I was becoming weaker and weaker, knowing that this was not going to sort itself out. The weight was falling off me. Why was nothing being done?

On day ten I was moved to ward 4B and was now under a new nursing team. I felt probably the lowest I had ever been. When the ward sister came in and introduced herself, she asked me how I was and I broke down. Emotionally I was gone and told her that I felt nothing had been done. It was probably the first time I had let my feelings show to anybody other than Linzi. The sister couldn't have been nicer and it really helped me that she listened to my concerns and was there for me. I rang Linzi in tears telling her how I could not carry on like this. Again she sorted out the boys, dropped them off at her parents' house and came straight to me. Linzi knew I wasn't in a good state but when she saw how upset I was in front of the sister it made her worry.

The sister organised for a doctor to come in and review me. From then on I felt like something was being done; tests started and procedures carried out. There was an outpatient's appointment at The Christie with Mark Saunders that I didn't want to miss. He was my specialist; I trusted him and I needed his opinion. After negotiations, Linzi was allowed to transport me from Whiston with a photocopy of my notes but I was to return straight back to the ward. I was very weak and could hardly walk. Dr Saunders explained that my only way forward would be to go on Total Parenteral Nutrition (TPN), basically to be fed artificially through a line. Could this be happening to me? I was a fit man, albeit with terminal cancer, but surely this wasn't my only option. Dr Saunders explained that he thought I wouldn't be able to eat solid food again. By that stage I was probably too weak to be upset. Linzi was emotional but she was also happy that this was an option.

She asked all the questions like, whether my hunger would be suppressed by the TPN and if I would be able to gain some weight whilst being fed this way. Having not eaten a thing for 10 days, only taking sips of water and having the odd bag of IV fluids, I was starving and had no energy to react. Dr Saunders took the details of the consultant I was under at Whiston and called him. He explained that there could be a funding issue with the TPN feed which we found to be ludicrous. That was the way it was; it was very expensive but I struggled with the fact that I could be denied funding for something that I needed in order to survive.

I returned back to the ward at Whiston and the ball was set in motion. A PICC line was inserted into my right arm and I waited for the feed to be organised. It was sanctioned, but for hospital use only, other things needed putting in place before I would be allowed to go home. In the meantime I changed consultants.

Mr Mike Scott, my old consultant from my playing days at Saints, was on his ward rounds and noticed that I was in. He popped in to see me and noticed a dramatic change in me from the last time he had treated me only a few months earlier for a previous obstruction. Mike agreed to take over my care and things started moving in the right direction. CT scans were organised and questions were asked about possible surgery to help my situation. Mike Scott contacted the pseudomyxoma specialists at The Christie and Basingstoke and forwarded my recent scans to them. Both specialist centres agreed to see me, but both said nothing more could be done for me. Both ruled out further surgery as it was deemed too dangerous, so there were no doors left open to me. Although I had started on TPN, I was still famished and my weight was still falling. As a result I was continuing to become weaker and was now unable to care for myself. Linzi was doing everything for me, getting me out of bed and taking me down to the shop. She would take me out in the wheelchair for fresh air and to get me away from the same four walls. I never thought I would see the day when I would be so dependent on somebody. Having been in hospital for three weeks I was desperate to get home. However, before this could happen I was transferred to Salford Royal's Intestinal Failure Unit, so they could assess me, sort out my nutritional requirements and train me how to administer the feed myself. This was easier said than done though because the IFU was in extreme demand. Mark Saunders and Mike Scott did their upmost to get me a bed. Between them they managed to do so.

In the ten days I spent waiting for a transfer I had a lot of time to think. What was I going to do if nobody was willing to take a chance on me and go back in? I knew that there was a big research campaign at The Christie to help find a cure for pseudomyxoma, but deep down I thought that this had come too late for me. It was my only hope though because there wasn't an option for an operation and the current forms of chemotherapy were not working for me. 'Did I have time to wait for the funding for this new ground breaking research?' I asked myself.

Scientists have used me as an example in the campaign, probably because of the fundraising I have done through the SPF which has helped towards the study – something I am very proud of – but possibly because I have defied the odds. It was a reality check to read in the appeal that people like me should only live for two to four years with this condition. It was seven years down the line; could I wait another two years for a possible cure? Probably not.

With this in mind I began doing my own research on the internet, just like I had done seven years previously when I was first diagnosed. Giving up was not an option and I refused to believe that nothing could be done for me. I began to explore possibilities, recalling what I was told back in 2006, specifically that the reason they could not cure me was because my small bowel was involved. This was also the reason for my current set back and it was preventing me from eating. So I asked myself, 'Why can't I have a bowel transplant?' After googling it I discovered that Oxford University Hospital carried out such a procedure. I asked the question to my consultants, none of which thought it would be feasible with my disease. It was worth a try, but now I had to try to get my head around being fed artificially through TPN. Hopefully, Salford Royal could sort out my nutrition and get me to a point where I could put back on some of the two stone in weight that I had lost whilst in Whiston Hospital. On May 13, 2013 I was transferred by ambulance to Salford Royal and they were great with me from the start. It was a very modern ward with great facilities. It was obvious from the outset that this team were experienced and specialised. I was hopeful that if anybody could help me this team would be able to and I was looking for hope.

As time progressed I realised that even with their expertise they could only help with the nutritional side of things. Nothing more could be done to help get my bowel working and, due to the tumours within my abdomen, I wasn't in a position to have a peg inserted into my stomach. My only hope of being able to eat again was dashed, so I would have to learn to get used to that idea. Although I was hungry, even sucking on a boiled sweet caused me pain.

A nasal gastro (NG) tube was inserted up my nose and into my stomach so that I could aspirate if I felt uncomfortable. Leaving the ward one day to go to a nearby hairdressers a number of people stared at me and checked out the nasal tube – that disturbed me. It gave me an insight into what disabled people must go through on a daily basis. It was hard and also very likely that I would have to have this on a permanent basis. How could I take my boys out with a tube up my nose and have people stare and point? The thought of this upset me.

I was told that the NG tube would be a permanent fixture, because this was my only way to get rid of the secretions in my stomach. I knew I wouldn't feel comfortable going out with it in, so figuring that if I put my mind to it, it could not be that hard, I asked if they could teach me how to insert them myself.

This way I could put one in when I felt the need to aspirate and also remove it when I needed to. I had struggled when the nurse had first inserted it as it is only natural to gag, but if I didn't want it in all of the time it was my only choice. From the reaction of the staff, I don't think this is commonly done, but after only one practice I mastered it and I found it easier being in control.

One morning on the ward rounds I asked the doctors again about the possibility of me having a bowel transplant. I was desperate and begged them to ask the question. It was a surprise when one explained that he was actually involved in some way with the transplant team in Oxford. He assured me that he would put my scans forward but made it very clear that he wasn't promising anything would come of it. All I wanted was the question to be asked so was happy and grateful that he would do that for me. Even though I knew it was a long shot, I was pleased. When I told Linzi about how I had almost pleaded with the team; she kept saying 'Don't build up your hopes.' Nevertheless, she was pleased that every avenue was being explored.

I was in Hope for a further four weeks and despite becoming mentally stronger I was physically weak and had not put any weight back on. The fact that I picked up a UTI just before I was about to be discharged didn't help and I was pretty poorly with that, hallucinating and spiking temperatures. It was a worrying few days for us because we didn't know what the problem was. After several tests it was discovered that the kidney stents that had been inserted a few months earlier had become infected. This resulted in an extra few days in hospital, but what was a couple of days when I had already been in for so long?

After 48 days I was finally discharged and was grateful to all the staff at the Intestinal Failure Unit at Salford Royal. The nursing staff had listened to me and helped me to become mentally stronger and had also been great with my family. All the time I was in there Linzi had been watching the aseptic protocol they use when connecting and disconnecting the TPN to my Hickman line. It is vital that this is carried out in a sterile way as the line sits so close to the heart and any infection could be very dangerous.

The staff answered any questions we had about this and were also great about the vast amount of visitors I had during my stay. This tough time made me realise what great friends I had and I was overwhelmed by how many made the effort to visit me. You realise that the friends you make through rugby are very special and although you go for long periods of time without contact you still hold that bond. In fact I was so lucky on the visitor front that the nursing staff became concerned I wasn't getting enough rest, but I loved having different faces each day to help me through. I thank every single visitor I had, especially the ones who travelled miles to come and see me.

I couldn't wait to get home to my newly renovated house that I had hardly spent any time in, but most of all I wanted to be back with my family and my boys. But at the same time going home was pretty scary because I felt a bit institutionalised. There were lots of changes to my life that I had to get used to with the biggest being the TPN and all that is associated with that. On the day of my discharge the homecare team, Baxter Healthcare, delivered a full sized fridge to my house, along with two weeks' worth of the nutritional feed (TPN). They also brought all the ancillary supplies I was going to need for the month. The amount of boxes was unbelievable. How were we going to manage to administer all of this?

At first the homecare team came to the house to connect and disconnect my feed. It was more complex than you would imagine. The fact that it is an aseptic procedure meant that Linzi would have to train properly. Each hospital has their own protocol and after speaking to the homecare nurses, it seemed like Salford Royal was the most difficult, but they pride themselves on a 0 per cent infection rate, so they must be doing something right. The least amount of people touching my line the better as this means there is less chance of infection, so we decided that Linzi would do the training and learn how to do it just in case I wasn't well enough to connect or disconnect myself. It didn't take her long before she was confident enough to go solo and soon the homecare team stopped coming unless we had a problem. I had to have an hour's worth of IV drugs through the line before disconnecting. Linzi drew them up and administered them but because she had to leave to go to work I began disconnecting myself once the IVs finished. Although it was hard at first, we got ourselves into a routine. Linzi was like my nurse, doing all the duties before she even left to go to work and then beginning again on an evening when it was time to connect me up. I knew she was under pressure, trying to make sure she was doing the best for me and making sure she was following the procedures correctly, but she just got on with it. She never moaned about it and I believe she would make a good nurse.

We had told both of the boys whilst I was still in hospital that I wasn't able to eat or drink again as we felt that we needed to be honest with them from the start. After all how can you hide the fact that I wouldn't be sitting down at the table to eat dinner or that I wouldn't be pinching their chocolate and sweets anymore? We had a long chat about how we should handle things with the boys and we decided that it was time for Taylor to know more about my illness. We did get some leaflets from the hospital to guide us but it wasn't going to be easy. In fact we dreaded the moment. Linzi was keen to get the timing right but it had to be done soon as he was about to start High School and he was approaching 12 years old. How long would it be before somebody asked him if his dad had cancer? We wanted him to be able to ask us questions instead of bottling his fears inside and becoming more worried. So one evening when he came into the kitchen/family room to get a snack, we were both sat on the settee whilst Koby was playing in his bedroom. I thought it was a perfect time, if ever there could be one. I hadn't discussed it with Linzi but just asked him to come and sit with us. It wasn't long before Linzi realised where the conversation was going and when I glanced over to her I could see she was fighting back the tears.

'You know I can't eat anymore don't you Tay?' I asked.

'Yes,' he replied.

'You do know that I'm not well, don't you?' He just nodded his head to reply.

Linzi put her arm around him. Staying strong and holding back her emotions, she asked, 'Do you know your dad has got pseudomyxoma?'

We knew he did know because we had talked openly about it, he knew I went for regular scans and checkups and obviously I had been in hospital on numerous occasions.

Linzi continued, 'Tay, do you know that pseudomyxoma is cancer?'

That was it, she had said the word. Taylor burst into tears and surprisingly said he didn't know. We actually thought that deep down he would have known from newspaper articles or TV interviews and so we were quite shocked. Linzi reassured him and we told him that I had had it for seven years, all of Koby's life. We highlighted all the challenges I had completed and how much I had achieved during that time. Taylor is a good boy, mature for his age and sensible. We asked him if he wanted to ask us anything or if he was worried about anything and reassured him that he could ask us or talk to us about anything. We told him that we wanted to be open with him now he was growing up and he soon composed himself.

Linzi had a little cry afterwards but to be honest I think we did okay. We both stayed strong and positive in front of Taylor and all credit to him, he took it well. It was a big relief for me as it had been on my mind for some time, but it was probably one of the hardest things we have had to do. You want to protect your children as much as you can but in these circumstances I believe we did the right thing.

Part 2

Linzi Takes Up the Story

28

The Call

Although the last seven years have been extremely difficult, we are grateful for the positives and thankful for the memories and good times we have shared together. Stephen has truly amazed me with his mental strength and the way he has overcome adversity by turning it into something positive.

The last few months have devastated me, watching Stephen deteriorate and seeing how weak he has become. It has broken my heart to see him crawling up the stairs on his hands and knees not having the energy to climb up them since he came home from Salford Royal. 'How long can he continue like this?' I asked myself. Although Stephen is not the type of person to give up, I was struggling to see how he could carry on fighting when nobody could give him any hope and it was obvious that the disease – pseudomyxoma – was catching up on him. Things didn't seem to be improving and with UTI after UTI, I could see he was on a downward spiral.

On Tuesday July 2, 2013 Stephen received a phone call, out of the blue from Mr Arun Abraham from the Intestinal Failure Unit at Salford Royal. He asked Stephen if we could attend a meeting with a surgeon from Oxford to discuss options following our request for a small bowel transplant. Of course we could attend, we were desperate for somebody to give Stephen some hope, but I was also very sceptical and worried in case it would set him back. Stephen has always needed confidence and without positivity he could lose focus, which had happened in the past. We were both very happy that somebody was giving up their time to travel all the way up north from Oxford to speak to us.

Stephen and I didn't really know what to expect or what would be said. I remember in the car on the way to the meeting saying to Stephen, 'Don't let it knock you back. You will be no worse off than you are now if they say there is nothing that can be done.' I kept thinking about the times when we met with the surgeons at The Christie and how that affected him mentally. Stephen had a good feeling about it though and repeatedly said, 'Why would somebody travel all that way just to tell me no?' I wanted to be as confident as him but I was frightened.

When we arrived at the ward I was even more apprehensive and nervous. We were asked to wait in the reception area. Arun joined us and we chatted whilst we waited. Stephen asked him his thoughts on the matter but he didn't give anything away. In fact he told us he didn't have any idea what the outcome would be. Before long, Arun received a call from the surgeon to say that he had arrived and so he went down to meet him. On his return he introduced us to Mr Anil Vaidya, Consultant Transplant Surgeon from Oxford's Churchill Hospital, and we were taken into a small meeting room.

My first impression of Mr Vaidya was that he was very calming, confident and casual. Dressed in jeans, trainers and a polo shirt, he was not the typical 'surgeon'. We both instantly liked him. After the initial introduction Mr Vaidya advised us that he knew our situation and that he had already looked at Stephen's scans. He then asked us to talk him through our journey. Stephen did most of the talking and he spoke from the heart, explaining what he had been through since the day he was diagnosed. Stephen described the way he had got himself to such a high level of fitness to now, where he was living on TPN, with no quality of life and without options to go forward. Stephen explained how he couldn't understand why nobody would take a chance, go back in and just clean up.

As we got him up to date, Anil crossed his legs, sat back and listened attentively to the details. He replied, 'How do you see yourself going forward with no options available to you?' Stephen explained that was the reason he had pushed so hard for this and for his scans to be sent on to the transplant team. What Anil said next was something neither of us expected or ever dreamed possible. In his relaxed, positive manner he explained, 'I am confident I can get you back to pre-2006 safely.'

Anil made it clear that this was his opinion, and said when he had put Stephen's case forward at an international conference only 50 per cent had a favourable view on that. He also explained that it had never been done before for somebody with pseudomyxoma and it would be a 'first in the world' operation. Anil immediately asked for a piece of paper and a pen and began to draw diagrams of the abdomen and the organs within. Both Stephen and I were in shock, neither of us looked up or even made eye contact with each other but instead listened intently to what was being explained. It all made sense, but it just wasn't sinking in. The more detail he went into, the more he filled us with positivity and overwhelming confidence. 'Where had this guy been?' I could tell in Stephen's voice that he had been given a massive lift. We asked several questions and all were answered instantly with reassurance. He blew us away. He told us to go away and think about it. He gave us his mobile number and his email address and told us to contact him anytime if we had any questions.

As we left the room, hand-in-hand we did not speak to each other. We were both in complete disbelief. Once we got into the car I said, 'Can you believe that?' I knew this is what Stephen had been searching for the last seven years; it was like he knew something was out there and that is why he didn't give up researching. Stephen just said, 'Oh my God, I've got to do that.'

'I know,' I replied. Stephen seemed shocked at my response. He knows I am always the one who thinks things are too good to be true but this time I had little doubt. Meeting Anil Vaidya on that day gave us a lifeline; he gave us the hope we needed with just that one encounter.

When we told family and friends, it was amazing. We were in tears and the hair on the back of my neck was standing up, but was it too good to be true? How come nobody else had suggested this?

The following day we sent an email to Anil to thank him for his consideration and offering Stephen a potentially life changing opportunity. We advised him that we were now in a position to request a slot in Oxford to have the necessary tests done to confirm suitability for the transplant.

Things moved very quickly and we were down at the Churchill Hospital, Oxford, the following Wednesday for 10 days whilst they put Stephen through the 'hoops' of assessments and whilst we met the team, including cardio thoracic, plastic surgeons, nutritionists and anaesthetists. Stephen had extensive bloods taken and underwent several tests and procedures including, chest x-rays, ultrasounds of the heart and liver, CT scans among others and thankfully got through them all positively.

There were a couple of results still outstanding when we left the hospital but they were going to take a week or so to be processed. It was now becoming a bit more real. We met a couple of bowel transplant patients during our stay, looking at how well they were, speaking to them about their journey and listening to how they, too, spoke so highly of Anil made our confidence grow even more. Although we had only spent a short time at the hospital, our trust in Anil and all members of the transplant team that we were lucky enough to meet was immense. I came away thinking that this dream could actually become a possibility. We now had something to work towards. We finally had some hope!

When we arrived home, it wasn't long before Stephen began to feel weak again. Surely he can't be getting another urine infection? He was showing all the same signs and his bloods confirmed it. By this time Stephen was getting fed up. He had had enough of feeling like this. It was becoming a pattern, one week of infection with a course of antibiotics and one week recovering on repeat. It was very obvious to me that it was getting him down. It was not like Stephen. He would come downstairs, get disconnected from his TPN, then just sit on the settee until it was time to be reconnected in the evening. He would then struggle up the stairs and go to bed. It was a far cry from the Stephen I know and I tried my best to motivate him. I didn't like seeing him like that and tried to explain that you feel more tired when you are not active. So I asked, 'Why don't you get on your turbo trainer?' or suggested we went for a walk round the block. He wanted to so badly, but he just couldn't muster up the energy which was so frustrating for him.

We were hitting a brick wall, finding no solution to the reoccurring infections. Stephen decided to ring The Christie urology department to ask them about the problem. They took down the details and said they would get back to him once they had spoken to the relevant doctors. Stephen couldn't wait and asked for my thoughts about contacting Anil in Oxford. He was hesitant as he thought it was a bit cheeky when Anil wasn't involved in the stent insertion but he was petrified of anything getting in the way of this dream. Anil had told us that we could call him anytime so we decided that it was our only option to get his opinion and advice. Stephen gave him a call. He needn't have been apprehensive as Anil was more than happy to listen and offer his help. He advised Stephen to wait for The Christie to get back to him and if they were unable to get him in soon for the stent removal, he would do it for him down in Oxford. The Christie had a waiting list so we took Anil up on his kind offer and travelled down to Oxford the following day. It was the final day of school before the summer holidays, so we gave the boys the option to come down to Oxford with us. Taylor, with his football commitments, decided to stay behind with my parents but Koby was quite keen to come down and spend a few days in a hotel.

We arrived late afternoon, checked into the guest house and admitted Stephen to the ward. Anil had contacted Stephen on our way down to inform him that everything was in place for the stent removal first thing the following morning, and that's what happened. After the procedure Anil came in and told us how the stents had become encrusted with infection and that it would not have been cleared without their removal. It was decided to see if Stephen could get by without the plastic stents, to try to keep him infection free in order for him to build his strength up for the major operation that potentially lay ahead. It was good for Koby to become familiar with the hospital, ward and staff if Stephen was going to be spending a long period of time there after the operation.

Whilst we were there the remaining outstanding results from the tests done during the work up came back. They showed that Stephen had zero antibodies in his blood, which meant that his sensitisation was as low as it could be, meaning that a match for transplant was more likely. That was another positive! All we had to do now was wait to see whether it was deemed feasible at the National Adult Small Intestinal Transplant (NASIT) meeting mid September 2013.

The stay in hospital lasted for 10 days and during that time I noticed that Stephen was becoming more fragile and less mobile, so much so that one day when we went into Oxford City for a look around, he bought himself a walking stick. I was shocked that he even suggested it and even more upset that he actually must have felt so bad that he needed it. It brought a tear to my eye watching him hobble with the stick, putting years on his age.

At the end of the 10 days, his blood levels finally came down to near normal and after completing the course of antibiotics and an ultrasound of his kidneys to check all was well, Stephen was discharged and we headed home.

The following day, Stephen's brother Neil was competing in the Bolton Iron Man in aid of the Steve Prescott Foundation. Stephen desperately wanted to go to support him as he knew how much hard work, time and effort had gone in to the training, but I feared he would not be strong enough. I also knew that if he didn't go he would feel defeated again by his illness and that would be another dent in his confidence. The weather was horrendous but in his true fighting spirit he made the decision to drag himself off the sofa. All four of us went along and tried to park as close as possible to the event route.

The new walking stick was a must and I could see that he was relying on it more and more. He didn't look well at all and I'm pretty sure he didn't feel well either but he put on a brave face and battled it out without a word. We anticipated spending an hour or so there, just enough time to show our support to Neil and his training partner John Bowes, who was also competing in aid of the Foundation. Instead, in true Stephen style he endured more than five hours and walked some distances to see them on different parts of the route. How he managed it I'll never know, but he never ceases to amaze me when he pushes his body to the limits. In this instance it was nowhere near what he had achieved before but one that probably impressed me the most as I could see how much effort he put in and how he really tested his mind and his body. This reassured me what a fighter he is and how mentally strong he was. I was very proud of both him and Neil that day.

The next day I'm sure Neil must have been aching after his achievements but I have to say Stephen also struggled to get out of bed. A far less achievement when it comes to physical strength, but right up there when you talk about mental strength. His now frail legs ached and the pain, where the tumour surrounded his stoma tortured him that day. I also ached, but mine was not a physical ache but an emotional one, watching Stephen suffer and endure such discomfort.

The pain only got worse for Stephen. The abdominal wall tumours were so raw and tender that they stopped him from sleeping. Frequently, I would hear him up during the night in the en suite trying to change his stoma bag just to get some relief. This was an effort in itself, taking both of us up to an hour as we had to incorporate all tumours. It was becoming harder to ease the pain and more and more ideas of dressing the area were failing as the disease was spreading to a wider vicinity. The pain for Stephen became unbearable and I could frequently see him wincing meaning the morphine was becoming more regular. It was like a vicious circle, the pain would keep him awake at night and the tiredness would make him lethargic during the day. What kind of life was he living? Not one that he would choose to live, I knew that.

As the days passed by, he busied himself preparing and perfecting his best man's speech for Martin Blondel's wedding. Martin is the General Manager of the Steve Prescott Foundation and a very close friend of ours. Stephen had used the time in Oxford to research and write the speech but he is a perfectionist and everything has to be done just so. He spent many hours reading over his speech and improving his power point. I was pleased he had a focus that week to help him to get through the pain barrier. It came to the night before the wedding and he began to complain that he didn't feel too good again. I know if he mentions something then he isn't good as he usually suffers a lot in silence.

I asked whether it could be nerves for the following day and he said it could be and took himself off for yet another early night hoping he would have a better day tomorrow, the wedding day. Unfortunately, during the night he became quite unwell, being sick and feeling generally ill. Initially, I put it down to pre-speech nerves but soon realised after the amount of aspiration from his NG tube that this was something more. Stephen is very good at knowing his own body and when he said he was texting Martin to let him know, I knew he doubted his presence at the wedding. For a split second I too thought it would be impossible for him to go, but then deep down I knew that there would be no way in the world he would let Martin and Karen down. I was right. He dragged himself out of bed and into his 'tails', leaving his NG tube in until the very last moment, continuously aspirating it. He so desperately needed a break from feeling like this, but it was out of my control and I felt so helpless. Again, Stephen did amazingly well. He made it through the day, pulling off a cracking speech and he was there to do all his duties as best man. I'm sure that people who didn't know what he was going through would not have known how bad he was feeling as he miraculously did not show on the outside how much he was suffering on the inside. I felt immensely proud of him and I know it meant the world to Martin and Karen to have him there. Stephen wasn't well enough to return to the evening reception. We went home after the speeches and by the time I had connected him to his TPN he had nothing left to give. He went straight to bed to rest. Although over the next couple of days he improved slightly, I still wasn't happy with the state of his health. When the district nurse phoned on the Monday to check how Stephen was getting on, I explained my concerns. Stephen was no doubt deteriorating and his pain needed reviewing. She agreed and suggested that the doctor from the hospice should make a home visit. This was arranged for the Wednesday morning.

Stephen's energy levels were non-existent. As he lay on the settee, I could see him getting frustrated. He was exhausted and I couldn't see how that was going improve if he didn't do anything to help. I can only imagine how difficult it is to motivate yourself to do something if you physically have nothing to give but I wanted to keep his spirits up. I was pushing him to keep mobile and encouraged him constantly. Admittedly, on some occasions, I was selfishly doing it for me as it was so hard to watch him like this. I suggested he tried to get on his turbo trainer and do some spinning just to get his legs going and more importantly, for me, his mind. He agreed but as I watched him struggle to get to the bike I could feel myself getting upset. This was not my husband, this was a frail man who was very poorly, but I could also see that he wasn't going to give up the fight.

He sat on the bike and managed to pedal for one mile. It took it out of him but I was so pleased that he had pushed himself to do something. His energy levels were so low that he couldn't lift his trailing leg over the bike to get off. It upset him because I had to help and think he felt so dependent on me because he needed more and more support. He sat back on the settee and stayed there for the rest of the day, not because he wanted to, but because he had no choice. He was too broken to do anything else – he couldn't carry on this way; it would gradually grind him down.

That evening after being connected to his TPN, as he tried to get up, his left leg gave way causing him to fall into the coffee table. His frustrations got the better of him and he broke down. 'I don't even have the energy to get up off the chair by myself; I cannot go on like this,' he cried. I helped him up and he hobbled, with his stick, up the stairs, as I followed carrying his drip stand and TPN. He went to bed. That was his life at the moment. Getting up, getting disconnected, sitting on the settee all day, getting reconnected and going to bed. What kind of quality of life is that for a 39 year old?

Dr Whittaker, the hospice doctor, came for the home visit the following day. It was early and I was still disconnecting Stephen. It had taken him longer to get up with the aches and pains resulting from the fall. His groin was very painful; he was frail and discontented.

Stephen explained all to Dr Whittaker, who asked him to lie on the sofa whilst he examined him and carried out the necessary tests. His temperature was up as was his heart rate and it wasn't long before Dr Whittaker told him it would be sensible to go into Whiston Hospital. After his previous few months, it was probably the last thing he wanted to hear but he was presenting early signs of sepsis.

Hospitals were becoming our second home but deep down we both knew that was where he had to be. Before we did anything, Stephen rang Anil. He wanted to keep him in the loop and to be honest we valued his opinion and expertise. He offered for us to go straight to Oxford, but Stephen didn't want to waste his or the team's time if he only needed antibiotics again. He decided he would go into Whiston, have the necessary tests and a decision would be made depending on the results. So bags were repacked and we set off for A & E. After several tests and bloods, it was confirmed that yet again Stephen was suffering from a serious infection. When you have a line in your body, it's the first thing you suspect as a primary cause. Because Stephen's Hickman line belonged to Hope Hospital, it meant Whiston were not allowed to touch it, going back to the protocols. So I had to arrange for a homecare nurse to come to the hospital to take blood cultures from the line in order to rule it out as a source of infection. All TPN would have to be stopped until the results of the cultures came back. No food, of course, means no energy so I was concerned about his nutrition as well as everything else.

In our mind, the likely cause of infection was another UTI because he had been so prone to them recently. They moved him from A & E to the assessment unit whilst we waited for the consultant. As we sat in the room, we knew the situation wasn't good. All we could think about was the transplant option and how we didn't want to jeopardise that chance. As we chatted and discussed whether or not to contact Anil again and take up his offer to go down to Oxford the consultant walked in. It was the same consultant who he had been under on his last visit before Mike Scott had taken over his care. The consultant, Stephen and I all remembered that time. I looked at Stephen and he looked at me and it didn't fill us with confidence as all those dark memories came flooding back. I knew instantly at that point where I wanted Stephen to be treated. There was no doubt in my mind that we needed to go to Oxford. Being away from home and away from the boys wasn't ideal but we needed Stephen to get the best possible care. To be fair, on this occasion the consultant did everything he could with regards to ordering all the tests. He actually said to the nurse that he owed it to this patient to do everything so as not to put his pending operation in danger.

Stephen was soon moved to a ward but instead of improving he seemed to deteriorate. He began to suffer severe back pain and his white cell count and CRP continued to rise. He had a rough night. The following day, Anil rang him to get an update. Quite quickly he told him that he needed to be down there so that he could treat him. As soon as he explained to Stephen that he was committed to his future care and that he needed to take over, we had no hesitation. An ambulance was arranged to transfer Stephen because he wasn't stable enough to travel by car. I rushed home, organised for the boys to stay at my parents' house, packed some clothes, Stephen's TPN and all the ancillaries needed and followed in the car.

When I arrived at the Churchill Hospital, Stephen had already been seen by Anil and was being assessed by the doctor. The plan was to get him down for an emergency CT scan to find out what was going on inside. A slot was provisionally booked for theatre just in case it was his kidneys, as suspected. It all seemed to happen very quickly. Stephen was taken for the scan at 10pm, less than three hours after he had been admitted. The results came back shortly after showing that his left kidney was obstructed and that he needed the stents inserting again as soon as possible. By midnight he was in theatre having the kidney drained and the stents put in. The speed at which he was treated confirmed that we had made the right decision to travel the 160 miles.

The following day Stephen was still in pain and his numbers were still very high, but we knew he was in good hands. We felt confident and safe here. We chatted long and hard and with the plan to put Stephen on the transplant list mid September, we decided that it was a sensible idea for Stephen to stay in the local area of Oxford until after the operation. We couldn't take the risk of going back home and him falling ill again. We spoke to Anil about it and he agreed that this was the right thing to do.

As the days went by, Stephen's back pain became more intense rather than improving and his bloods still showed high infection levels. The medical team began to explore other possible causes. The kidneys were looking okay, as was their function, so could it be something else?

After reviewing his scans the transplant doctors noticed that Stephen had a large abscess within his psoas muscle. The cause was unknown. It was arranged for Stephen to go back down to radiology in order for them to put in a pig tail drain through his back into the muscle guided by CT scan. Whilst down at the scanner Stephen asked what might have caused the abscess and he was told that one of the possible causes could be a perforated bowel. We both went into immediate panic mode. We instantly remembered being told at the work up that a perforated bowel could mean no transplant. We were reassured that you are usually very sick and much more unwell than what Stephen was presenting, but it was still a possibility. Stephen was good at disguising how ill he was because he would just keep fighting on and this was in the back of my mind. It was like being on a rollercoaster; our emotions were all over the place. One minute we were excited and full of hope of a transplant and the next we were petrified that something was going to stand in the way and rule it out. It felt like I had the weight of the world on my shoulders at times and it was a very stressful time for us both. The procedure was very painful for Stephen but hopefully it would release some of the pressure and ease the terrible pain he had been suffering once the drain started to work. For Stephen, the pain only increased. He could no longer lie or sit properly as he had a tube sticking out of his back. He couldn't get comfortable. We tried propping him up at all sorts of angles but he was struggling. Overnight, the drain didn't do much and it was agreed that it would possibly need a larger drain inserting. The thought of it made Stephen grimace as he knew what lay ahead. He was taken back down to CT. While he was down there having the larger drain inserted, they decided to investigate the root cause. They inserted some contrast to determine the origin. It wasn't good news. It was a perforated bowel. When Stephen came back to the ward I could tell by his face that something wasn't right. I asked him how it had gone; he just shook his head and said, 'I'll tell you in a minute.' As the porters left the room, I could see his eyes filling up. 'This could be dream over,' he said. Anil came into see us, he had looked at the scans and once again in his confident, casual manner he explained that these results wouldn't change any plans he had. Whether or not he was having doubts inside, he didn't show it and he put our minds at rest, explaining that because the bowel had perforated into the muscle, they were able to give it a way out of the body through the drain. Another big sigh of relief! Although things were going wrong and hurdles were thrown at us, we felt very lucky that positives followed.

Stephen was very uncomfortable and it was hard to see him that way, I again felt useless. His mobility was now enormously reduced and he could not use his left leg. This had been since his fall back home, but with new light on the situation it was more than likely caused by the abscess in the muscle as it is linked to that area. Also on the scans it was identified that the tumours inside were pressing on the femoral nerve, also causing limited mobility and sensation in his left leg. He was the weakest I had ever seen him, mentally and physically, at this point. He was deteriorating before my eyes; I could see that even though I was with him 14 hours a day. I knew he was in the best possible hands but the dream of the transplant was drifting away. We both tried to remain positive and Stephen remained motivated but the stress of being away from home, our boys and things not going smoothly were taking their toll. Stephen became very emotional and would quite often open up and get upset, which was not usual for him. I tried to be strong for him and reassure him but at times I needed reassuring myself.

We were very lucky that family and friends continued to visit, even though we were so far away. For that we were totally grateful, knowing we had a great support network. We also became good friends with a couple of fellow transplant patients and their families. Curtis and Susie had very similar circumstances to us as their girls were similar ages to our boys. Curtis also had a multi visceral transplant and was probably the most similar case to Stephen's.

It was always good to talk with them and share emotions and feelings. I was sharing the transplant flat with Corrina, whose partner, Ian had just had a bowel transplant and we became close. When you share something so special you build up a strong connection and that's what happened. When Ian left the ward he too moved into the transplant flat so they could stay local for his after care. They used to visit us on the ward on a daily basis and Stephen used this time to ask the questions he needed answering from a patient's point of view. It was good for Stephen to see how well all the previous bowel transplant patients were doing. It inspired him to keep up his fight.

We also had a surprise visit from Mr Tom Cecil, Stephen's surgeon from Basingstoke. We hadn't had much direct contact with him since early 2007 when he had transferred us to the care of The Christie oncology team. We had requested him to look at scans during the following years and ask for his opinion but that was done through the consultants. It was great to see him again, he had given us so much hope back in 2006 and we still thought very highly of him. Anil had been in touch with him to further his understanding of pseudomyxoma and he was keen to come and meet with Stephen again before the transplant as he hoped to be involved. He confirmed to us that there was nothing more he could do for Stephen and that he was excited that a new door may be opened through Stephen's bravery. He also expressed his confidence in Anil after their meetings and he thanked Stephen for taking the big step into the unknown not only to benefit himself but hopefully lead the way for other PMP sufferers. It was good to know that he was onboard and it was good to see him again.

Stephen and I spent long hours together day after day and it brought us really close. It gave us chance to edit the book and also spend quality time together. We have always been very close; especially since the diagnosis, we make a good team and this time together reinforced our relationship.

Lying in bed and not being mobile was not only frustrating for Stephen but also made him vulnerable to chest infections. He had fluid on one lung and infection on the other. Anil told me one day to buy him some balloons. He told Stephen to keep blowing them up to keep his lungs working. Stephen liked being given targets and although he found it difficult at first, once he managed to do one, he continued blowing them up. It was hard work for him, so instead of blowing them up, releasing them and blowing them up again, he tied every one he inflated so that Anil could see his efforts. His room resembled a child's birthday party.

Stephen seemed to have two or three good days and then he would get another setback. The team could see how frustrated he was getting, lying on the bed, in lots of pain from the back drain and the abdominal wall tumours, and unable to walk due to the left leg problem. He was also now connected to his TPN 24 hours a day, seven days a week due to erratic blood sugars which made it harder for him to get about. Anil arranged for a physio to come and see him and to bring him an exercise bike to his room. This would not only help his lungs, but also his fitness level. He needed to be fit for the major operation.

The bike was a great idea for Stephen. It helped him mentally as much as it did physically. The physio brought it one Saturday afternoon when I had taken the boys and my parents into Oxford whilst they were visiting. Taylor received a text from Stephen to tell him he had managed to do 5K on the bike. I was delighted, as he looked too weak to even get out of bed when we left him. So he continued to do his 5K each day, and considering how bad his health was everybody was shocked. He slowly began to increase his mileage and by the following week he was clocking up to 15K a day. I could see how pleased he was and he was keen to do more. It gave him a boost he needed but it was a double edged sword because although it was helping his fitness, his lungs and his mind, the dieticians were struggling to get enough calories in his artificial feed to keep up with the calories he was burning during the exercise and therefore he would not maintain his weight, which was already well below his usual weight. It was important to get a balance, so the dietician, Marion asked him to hold back, not stop but keep it to a maximum of 5K a day. It was hard for Stephen as he just wanted to keep going and get himself as fit as he could be for the operation. This was his only way of exercising as he was unable to walk with all his other problems. I think he wanted to prove to the consultants that he was still suitable for the transplant even though so much had changed since his work up. Anil and the team wanted to get him on the list as soon as possible. They could see the changes in him and were aware of all the complications being thrown at him. It was agreed that Stephen's case would be put forward for approval at a transplant meeting in Manchester on September 9. We were asked to put together a testimonial letter to be read out at the meeting, giving Stephen's point of view of why he should be suitable and also acknowledging the risks associated.

The outcome of the meeting was positive and after dotting the I's and crossing the T's, we were given the green light to go officially on the transplant list. Paperwork had to be completed and on Friday, September 13 we were informed that he was now live on the database and active on the transplant list. We were both absolutely delighted. It was now really happening.

I think we thought the call was going to come straight away. Every evening when I left him at the hospital I thought I might get a call during the night. I was on edge all the time I was away from him. I'm not sure why but I always presumed the call would come in the early hours of the morning, so when I woke each morning I initially felt disappointed that we hadn't heard anything.

After the first week that pressure eased and we became more patient, although it was always in our thoughts and conversations. Our lives revolved around it and that feeling was increased by staring at the same four walls all day every day, waiting. We were excited at this chance and gradually becoming desperate but we took each day as it came. Each time we saw Anil we would ask him if he had received any offers. He would always tell us if he had and explain the reasons of their unsuitability. We knew that the offer had to be perfect to give Stephen the best chance but we also liked being reassured that the offers were coming in even if they weren't right for us.

I don't think anybody can imagine the feelings you experience unless you have been in that situation. The feelings of hope, excitement, nervousness and desperation were mixed with feelings of guilt at being so desperate. For Stephen to get his dream meant that somebody else would lose their life and their family would be suffering. It was very strange but I don't think you can dwell on it too much. Transplantation is such a gift and we felt extremely grateful to be lucky enough to be on the list.

During the wait, Stephen became unwell again and his bloods showed another infection. After several tests, results showed that his kidneys had become blocked again. So this meant another trip to theatre for stent replacements. It was one thing after another but he continued to bounce back and motivate himself to carry on when most people would have given up. He was soon back on track and back on his bike. He also started doing some very light hand weights to build up some of the muscle he had lost in his arms. He strapped light weights to his ankles and tried to get his leg muscles working too. He tried everything to help himself. After doing the ankle weights his left leg began to swell. At first he put it down to doing too much, but as the days went on it became apparent it was something a little bit more serious. It turned out to be a blood clot from his groin to his knee. He was taken down to radiology to have a filter inserted but unfortunately, they discovered that it was the tumour causing the clot so the filter would get easily overrun and therefore the filter wouldn't be worthwhile. It was decided that they would leave him until he got the call for surgery and then take him down and do the procedure just prior to going to theatre.

It was very difficult for Stephen as not only had he been dealing with all the hiccups, constant pain and stuck in a room staring at the same four walls, he was conscious that he was missing out on time with the boys. He missed going to watch Taylor play football, he also missed both boys' birthdays and their first days back at school after the summer, which was made even more difficult as Taylor started high school which is quite a big deal. I was able to go home for these important dates but he couldn't. We were very thankful for Skype as we were able to see them every night and talk with them about what they had done during that day which we used to look forward to and it really helped us feel closer to them.

From the day Stephen went active on the list I also remained in Oxford on a permanent basis, with no home visits. I didn't want to travel back up north in case he got the call so I made a decision to stay. It wasn't an easy choice. As a mum it is so hard to be away from your children, but at the same time I knew what was important at that time. The boys were fine, they were being well looked after by my parents and they were being kept in a routine. They knew they could call us at anytime, we were always on the other end of the phone or they had their ipads and could Skype us as they pleased. Taylor would tell us about his football training and Koby would talk us through his school day, that's if he wasn't too busy watching *Coronation Street*. He told us on several occasions that he didn't have time to chat, which deep down hurt as it was our only contact with him, but on the other hand we found it comforting to know that he was happy and secure and obviously not missing us like we were missing him. Taylor is older and understands our feelings more; he always made time to talk to us. Koby was keen to talk if he had something exciting to tell us or if he had made something he wanted to show us. On one occasion he had drawn a picture in school. It was of Stephen on the operating table, with the surgeon, Anil, standing over him with a knife, dripping with blood. At the side he had drawn a table with three organs on, a small bowel, stomach and pancreas. This made us laugh. We joked that it was a good job the school were fully informed of what was happening or they may have classed this as 'strange behaviour'! It also made us realise that, although Koby is only seven years old, he had fully taken on board what was planned and obviously understood to a certain extent. The boys seemed to be taking it all in their stride which made the pain of being apart easier for us to deal with.

The longer we spent in the hospital, the more obsessed I became with looking at the monitors. Stephen used to tell me to stop looking, as if things didn't appear to look as they should I would begin to worry, often unnecessarily. On Monday, September 30, I could see from his obs that things weren't looking great and that his saturation levels were decreasing. Stephen was also drifting off to sleep during the day which wasn't like him. He was sent down for a chest x-ray which confirmed that he had an infection on his right lung again and he was put back on a nasal cannula for support.

I received a phone call at 3am. Before I even answered it I knew that it wasn't the going to be 'the call' the one we had been waiting for. I answered in anticipation; it was the nurse from the ward explaining to me that Stephen was very poorly. His oxygen levels were concerning and the ICU doctors were assessing him so that he could be transferred into Intensive Care. I quickly got dressed and ran over to the hospital. Luckily, I was onsite at the hospital flat, which had become my home for the last few months, so I was only minutes away.

I was shocked when I first saw Stephen, there was a noticeable deterioration from when I had left only hours earlier. He was slumped in his bed on maximum oxygen support available on the ward and his numbers didn't look good! He was exhausted and drowsy but still able to communicate. He took his oxygen mask off, only to tell me he was okay and not to worry! The nursing staff stayed in his room whilst arrangements were being made for his move to ICU. Seeing him like this frightened me. I began to realise that the transplant may now be too late. This was serious. The logistics of being so far away from home meant that it wasn't worth me contacting family and friends. It would only cause them concern at this hour and there was nothing they could do. I decided I would wait until I knew more before worrying them during the night. I was pleased that we had managed to build up good relationships with the staff during our stay and I relied on them for support. I had to be strong for Stephen. I knew that he always looked at my reaction to things so I couldn't just fall apart and panic.

When Stephen was taken through to ICU I was asked to wait in a side room whilst they assessed him. It seemed to take forever. I didn't like being away from him, I felt even more out of control not knowing what was happening and the nerves kicked in.

The ICU consultant came in and spoke to me. He warned me that Stephen was requiring the maximum amount of high flow oxygen available to him and if things didn't improve he would have to be put on a ventilator. I could see other patients on the unit with the same thing and it didn't look good. I was scared. Would he ever recover from this? Stephen had never been in intensive care before apart from immediately after his last surgery, but that was a planned visit so it really hit home how ill he had become.

The consultant agreed to see how he coped before taking these desperate measures but he wasn't confident that he would escape being ventilated.

When I saw Stephen again, he looked surprisingly much improved. The extra support given on this unit had obviously helped with his oxygenation and he was much more alert. He kept telling me that he didn't need to be on this ward and that he felt like a fraud taking up a specialist bed, but that was just Stephen, he obviously needed to be there as he was much sicker than he thought.

As a last ditch attempt not to put him on a ventilator, the physio explained that he could try a 'hood'. It looked like an astronaut's mask which was sealed over his head with lots of wires attached. It was very claustrophobic and he was told that not many people can tolerate it for long periods of time, but he was willing to give it a go if it meant not having to be ventilated. He didn't like the hood, but he managed it for short spells just to boost his oxygen levels. His spirits were still high and I remember him asking me to take his photograph and him sending it to friends in a text saying, 'Next challenge, the moon!' He wasn't beaten yet!

I think the nurses on the ward were surprised at how Stephen got over this set back. He seemed to improve quite quickly, against the odds, and his oxygen requirements started to reduce. Stephen worked hard with the physios and was very motivated to do the exercises given to him to help improve his lung function. After a couple of days he asked if they could bring his exercise bike from the ward into the ICU so he could continue working his legs. The physio also got him up walking, something he hadn't done much of since he got the blood clot. It was good to see and it wasn't long before he was in a position to be moved back to the ward. It was quite amazing how he turned things around. He obviously had excellent care but his own mind set played a big part in his speedy recovery. I could tell that from the reactions he got from the ICU staff.

Stephen was glad to be back on the ward and back in his own room as it could get quite noisy on the intensive care unit and he was tired. We were back to waiting again for the all-important call. The days became longer but I encouraged Stephen to continue to walk as he had in ICU with the physio. We would do a lap of the ward each day which slowly increased as the days went by. Stephen was reluctant, he found it difficult and he had his TPN to push too, but he did it. He also continued with his bike, he enjoyed this much more than the walking. To motivate him to walk to increase the strength in his legs and his core I used to 'trade off' with him. If he would walk a lap or two, I would help him with writing the book as it was so close to completion and he was desperate to get it finished. I wasn't so keen to help him as I didn't want to have to relive all the memories of the journey we had been on.

As the days went by we began to think the call was never going to come. Then an offer came from a B+ donor. Perfect! Unfortunately, the family did not consent to the bowel. We totally understood and had absolutely no resentment; however we were disappointed as we knew it could be a while before another B+ donor became available with it being such a rare blood group. Later that day, Stephen's oxygen requirements increased and he was put back on a nasal cannula, his bloods also showed some kind of yeast infection. Every day was becoming a battle.

The following morning I had a phone call from Koby. He wasn't very well and he was staying off school. He sounded unusually quiet and I felt very guilty about not being there for him. I became upset because when children are ill they only want their mum. Although I knew my mum and dad were doing a great job with both of the boys and they were getting lots of love and attention, everything changes when they are not well. I needed to be at home. Stephen begged me to go back, which made me even more upset. What if he got the call? That would be just our luck. He repeatedly told me, 'Nothing is going to happen here, I'm not going to get the call, just go home and be with the boys for a couple of days'. Stephen knew how hard it was for me to be apart from them, after all he felt the same. I seriously thought about going, but Stephen was having his PICC lines removed due to the yeast infection and I wanted to be around for that. The specialist line nurse was familiar with us, as were most of the staff, as we had been there for so long. She asked me about the boys, but I was so emotional that I began to cry in front of her. That was unusual for me and Stephen once again told me to go home. I was probably annoying him a bit by not going as he desperately wanted to ease my guilt. When Stephen went down for a further chest x-ray, I decided to get a break away from the hospital and go back to the flat. This was very rare for me as I was happy to spend all my time there, but things were just catching up with me. I hadn't been there long when Stephen phoned me to say we had some unexpected visitors. Friends Paul Barrow and Terry Flanagan had called in on their way home from a business meeting, so I made my way back over to the hospital to see them.

On my way, I saw Anil on the corridor. He waited for me to catch him up. He asked how I was and quickly went on to tell me that Stephen had an offer. Initially, I presumed it was the same as all the others, unsuitable, until Anil continued to say it was a very good offer. I asked him if he was going to accept it and he told me that he was. It was hard to take in. Why was I surprised? We had been waiting for this call for so long, yet it came when I was least expecting it. I explained how I had very nearly made the trip back up north to be with Koby. He was just about to go in and tell Stephen. Paul and Terry were in with Stephen, who introduced them to Anil and there was a bit of general chat. I was looking at Anil, waiting for him to tell him but he waited a couple of minutes. I had a big grin on my face and was bursting with excitement. Then Anil casually asked, 'Well are you ready?'

Stephen said 'Yes,' not really knowing what he was asking.

'Are you ready, ready?' asked Anil.

I then had to spell it out, 'You've got an offer, it's happening,' I said with tears in my eyes and a huge smile on my face.

Once Stephen had digested the news he beamed, 'Bring it on!' Paul and Terry were also delighted but I think they felt a little intrusive as it was quite an emotional moment. They decided to go and grab a coffee whilst Anil talked us through the next steps.

It was really happening!

29

Theatre of Dreams

I don't think I have ever experienced such a vast mixture of feelings all at the same time as I did on October 15, 2013 – and I doubt I ever will again.

I was overwhelmed, bursting with happiness and excitement that the time we had dreamt about had finally arrived. At the same time I was also nervous, scared and frightened of what lay ahead.

The time from 6.40pm, when we learnt of the offer of a suitable donor, to 10pm when Stephen finally went to theatre moved very quickly. During that short time a lot of things had to be organised and carried out. It was a good thing that we didn't really have a lot of time to dwell on what was actually happening.

After the initial shock of the news, we began to make phone calls to our family and closest friends to let them know the time had come. It was very emotional and each time I had to tell somebody I had to fight back the tears. They were tears of joy, I think, but to be honest I can't say for sure. Although we wanted this so badly we were also fully aware of the massive risks attached to such a procedure. Most of our family and friends just felt elated for us because they knew how desperate we had become and that the benefits outweighed the risks tenfold. As I was making calls myself, I could hear Stephen in the background calling some of his closest friends. The snippets I was hearing were heart-wrenching and he was obviously preparing in case the unthinkable happened. He thanked them for their friendship, for being there for him and for all that they had done over the years. It was hard for me to concentrate on what I was saying on the other phone as I just wanted to hold him and tell him that everything was going to be okay. Don't get me wrong, we were both extremely positive and confident and we wanted it more than anything in the world. But I just can't imagine, no matter how hard I try, what must have been going on in Stephen's mind at this time. He did go a little bit quiet for a short period, but with nurses in and out getting him prepared he had no choice but to focus his energy on the surgery.

Bloods were taken, as was an ECG, and then he was quickly whisked down to radiology where a team had been on standby to insert a filter in order to prevent the blood clot in his left leg from travelling upwards towards his lungs.

The procedure took about an hour. During that time I had a lot of time to think and my thoughts went to the donor's family and what they must have been going through. Our emotions couldn't have been anymore contrasted. I felt very sad for them and the tragic circumstances for that one family were going round in my head. Could they ever know the lifeline they were giving to Stephen and to us as a family? We were extremely grateful to them for their willingness to agree to the gift of organ donation. I put myself in their shoes. Would I have done the same? It emphasised to me how important it is to carry a donor card and to make your family aware of your wishes. Without this offer of life I'm pretty sure Stephen would not have survived much longer. In Oxford we all knew that time was running out for him. I wonder if the family of the donor would ever understand what a difference they made to us. Also during this time I spoke with Anil and he tried to prepare me for how long Stephen maybe down in theatre, although this was unknown as it had never been done before, he estimated that the surgery would be over 24 hours long. He explained that they would get Stephen into the operating room as quickly as they could, so that they could begin the tumour removal sooner rather than later, as nobody could predict how long it would take. As always Anil appeared very calm, although I'm sure inside he too must have had some apprehension, nerves and maybe some excitement, after all this was pioneering surgery. He also asked me if we could try to keep the details out of the public domain. We had already had several conversations with him about this during the weeks leading up to this point. We knew we had to protect the donor's family and also with it being the first time surgery of this kind that had been carried out, the team wanted Stephen back on the road to recovery, eating and drinking again before details were released. This suited us as family as we too wanted to keep it a private matter.

Once Stephen was back in his room on the ward, we were given time to Skype the boys. We had talked and discussed how we would play this over and over in the time we had been waiting and we didn't know what was the right or wrong choice but Stephen desperately wanted to see and speak to the them which was only to be expected with what he was about to endure.

At the beginning of the call, both of the boys were jumping up and down. After all, this is what we had been waiting for but it didn't take Taylor long to realise the seriousness of what was about to happen. His face soon changed as did his actions. He quickly became quiet as Stephen stressed how much he loved them both and how proud he was of them. Stephen began to get upset which in turn brought tears for both me and Taylor. It was very emotional. I just wanted to be able to give them all a big hug but with the boys being so far away it was impossible. Koby showed his innocence and could not understand why we were reacting in this way; he was unaware of the potential consequences of such a risky operation. He proceeded to ask, 'What is wrong with you all? You should be happy!' We were all happy and although we managed to compose ourselves and end the call on a positive note, I still felt emotionally drained. Stephen and Taylor shared some texts, which showed Taylor's maturity.

Taylor Prescott: 15/10/2013 21:06:00
Good luck dad we're all saying prayers love you so much xxx

Steve: 15/10/2013 21:14:21
Taylor u have made me so proud 2 b your dad. Your dedication to your football is fantastic.
U r halfway there to completing that promise you made me a long time ago.
If you keep going, keep on trying and never give up, like I didn't you're sure to b a champion!

I love u so much mate, that no one can take that away from us. Take care and keep on with your positive attitude.
I love u dad. Xxx

Taylor Prescott: 15/10/2013 21:22:27
Thank you so much that has got me in tears with happiness I love u so much keep fighting xxxx

I had always been so positive but I realised how risky this procedure was, especially with Stephen's lungs being a problem and I began to imagine how hard the next few days would be.

Dr Dyer, who had looked after Stephen in ICU a couple of weeks earlier came in to see us, also the nurses from the ward came to tell us how pleased they were for us that the perfect offer had finally arrived. Soon the negative thoughts disappeared and the excitement started to kick in again.

I saw Anil in the corridor. He told me that Stephen would be going down earlier than first thought. They were now aiming for 10pm as opposed to midnight as originally thought. Stephen's brother, Neil, and his wife, Jill, had already started their journey from St Helens but with the start time being brought forward it was unlikely that they would make it in time to see Stephen before he went to theatre. However they would be there to support me through the long hours that lay ahead.

In what seemed like no time, the theatre porters arrived and I was able to accompany Stephen right into the anaesthetic room as I had done on his previous surgery in 2006. It was very different this time. The mood was much better, more relaxed in fact. Stephen was having a joke with the anaesthetist as they prepared to put him to sleep. Stephen was not frightened as such, or at least he didn't show it and I felt surprisingly okay too. Strange, considering what lay ahead, but I think the confidence we had in the team was overwhelming, we had built up good personal relationships with them and we trusted them. Also Stephen wanted this so badly, we both did. We knew this was his only option and if anybody could give him this lifeline it was this team.

I was given the nod that it was time to leave, so I gave him a kiss, said what I had to say to him and I left him with a smile on his face. I wasn't even upset as I left the theatre; I was feeling positive and happy. I did have butterflies, but I couldn't work out whether they were down to nerves or excitement.

By the time I walked back to the ward to collect some of Stephen's personal belongings I received a call from Neil and Jill to say they had arrived. They had only missed him by 15 minutes. They had brought down the very same medal that he had taken down to theatre with him in Basingstoke. I am not superstitious but I also didn't want to tempt fate, so I asked one of the transplant nurses off the ward if she would take it into theatre to him. Although I knew he would already be asleep it was comforting to know he had it with him. They taped it to his pillow at the side of his head.

Neil, Jill and I took our seats in the relatives' room opposite the theatre. This is where we would spend the duration of the operation. I think Neil and Jill had expected me to be in a bit of a state during this time. I also expected myself to be in a state, but I think the adrenaline had kicked in and I was actually quite calm. I know deep down I was nervous as I was noticeably shaking and I was also physically sick on several occasions during that night, but on the exterior I was calm and confident. I surprised myself! Neil on the other hand, paced up and down a fair bit before settling to a certain extent.

We knew we were in for a long night. Every door that creaked and every footstep we heard made us edgy. I was constantly looking over my shoulder at the glass panel in the door. After about the first four hours we had every noise down to a tee. Jill and I would look at each other and say, 'That was the lift' or, 'That's the automatic doors to ICU'. In the end it became a bit of a joke. Neil managed to get some sleep on the pull out bed, but Jill and I chatted the whole night, wondering how things were going and waiting for some news.

At 5am I received a phone call from Anil. He explained that the first part of the surgery had gone well. They had removed the organs and the tumour successfully. He explained that Stephen had been stable throughout. However, there was a 'but' because the new organs had been delayed due to a problem with the heart recipient. This meant that they weren't expecting them to arrive until much later that day so Stephen had to be kept under anaesthetic and in the operating theatre during this time. Obviously, this wasn't ideal but the fact that Anil had said he had removed the tumour overshadowed everything else. Wow! I don't think we could have asked for anything more at this point. The first part of the surgery had taken far less time than I had anticipated and I was delighted.

Not long after the call from Anil, Tom Cecil also rang me. He was very pleased with how things had gone so far. He explained that they had packed Stephens abdomen whilst he waited but he remained stable and he suggested the break in surgery would be good for Stephen.

We waited for Stephen's parents to arrive. We knew they were leaving St Helens early and we couldn't wait to fill them in on the updates we had received. We were really excited. I didn't feel tired at all even though I had not had any sleep; I was on a high. The nerves I had the previous night seemed to get less and less. I had a really good feeling that everything was going to be alright. I think part of the nerves was fear that they would open Stephen up and decide that they couldn't do anything for him, now that those fears were over I was fairly relaxed.

Pat and Eric arrived, we all just stayed in the relatives' room, chatted and appeared to be normal, not like when we were in Basingstoke seven years previously, although we still flinched every time the door went or the phone rang.

I received a text from Anil mid morning to say that Stephen was still stable and that they were still waiting for the organs. Just to get little updates like that helped me stay calm and relaxed. Half of the time it is the not knowing that makes it hard. I was extremely grateful for the updates.

Corrina and Ian, whom I had been sharing the intestinal transplant flat with, came in to visit us and to see how things were progressing as did Susie and Curtis, who were back at clinic for a follow up that day. It was great to chat with them all and it helped to pass the time. I was glad that Neil and Jill and Pat and Eric got the chance to meet them too as they were living proof that this operation can change your life around. Anil also came in to see us and to reassure us that Stephen was doing okay despite the long, unexpected wait. He seemed pleased with how Stephen was coping and reaffirmed that he had been 'rock stable' throughout. He advised that the organs were due to arrive at the hospital at 4:35pm.

I was absolutely fine until that time approached and then I started to feel nervous again. I left the relatives room and began pacing the corridors outside, looking through the windows to see if I could see the organs arriving. There was no sign of them. I began to imagine that there was a big problem. What if they didn't come? What would happen then? Stephen was opened up with basically no insides. I started to get nervous and the sickness set in again. I remember seeing Anil and Professor Friend going back into theatre. It was now 5pm. I asked them where the organs were. They had been delayed further and weren't expected until approximately 6pm. I just couldn't settle. This was probably the hardest part ... waiting.

I saw Tom Cecil going back to theatre and I asked him if there was any news on the organs. He said the same as Anil and added that they would be starting doing some more work on Stephen now in preparation for the arrival.

At 6.35pm, the organs finally arrived. I spoke to one of the surgeons who had been to retrieve them. He confirmed that the organs were now in theatre and that they were in pristine condition. A big sigh of relief came from me and the nerves quickly settled again. I knew we were in for another long night, but I was happy. We were back on track!

Jill and I returned to the relatives' room where Pat, Eric and Neil were still waiting. We updated them and we all felt much more relaxed. We hadn't moved all day and we were getting hungry. We decided that we would order a takeaway to be delivered to the hospital. That was probably the first thing I had managed to eat since Stephen had received the call about the donor more than 24 hours previously. It felt strange that we were having a Chinese whilst Stephen was across the corridor having major surgery and we did joke about it at the time but we were happy that things were going well.

Stephen's parents left shortly after as they had booked a hotel for the evening. Neil, Jill and I prepared to stay another night in the relatives' room. At 10pm, much sooner than we imagined, Anil and Tom Cecil both appeared at the door. My heart sank. I didn't expect both surgeons to be giving an update and I immediately assumed there was a problem. I quickly made my way to the door and as soon as I saw their faces I knew everything was okay. They were both smiling and eager to update us.

The second part of the operation was now complete. Stephen now had a new stomach, pancreas and bowel. The surgeons seemed very happy with how it was going; Stephen had remained stable throughout and was over another hurdle. Tom's job in surgery was over; however Anil was going back into theatre to work alongside Henk Giele and the plastic surgery team who now had the task of transplanting the abdominal wall. I was advised that this could take up to a further ten hours. I felt elated with how things were progressing and was so pleased that the new organs were all in place.

I felt confident enough to nip back over to the flat for a shower and a change of clothes. This was the first time I had left the corridor since Stephen went into theatre but I was happy. Jill came across to the flat with me and Neil stayed in the relatives' room in case of any new updates.

When we got back to the hospital we spent another night chatting. I felt much less anxious and was feeling excited for the future.

To be honest the time went quite quickly and it wasn't long before we had another visit from Anil. He came in at 4.35am with the final update. It was all done, tumour removed, new organs in and abdominal wall transplant complete! What more could we ask for?

Anil was very happy and so was I. He showed me some photographs of Stephen on the operating table, one before they had begun the marathon surgery and one as he looked now. I was absolutely amazed by what they had achieved. I knew from looking at what they had done that Stephen was going to be delighted. It was so much more than we could have ever hoped for. The tumour that had perforated his skin was all gone as was the tumour within. It was like a miracle. I was so excited to see Stephen and his reaction to the results but I had to wait for them to get him settled in ICU.

I knew we still had a very long way to go, but after 32 hours of surgery he had the worst out of the way and he was now on the road to recovery.

Words cannot express how grateful I was to the whole team who had worked so hard to give us this lifeline and the chance of a much better quality of life. They had given Stephen his dream.

I couldn't wait to share the news with Stephen and tell him that he had done it. He had beaten pseudomyxoma peritonei!

'What the mind believes the body achieves!'

Part 3

Postscript by Mr Anil Vaidya, Consultant Transplant Surgeon from Oxford's Churchill Hospital

Stephen Prescott: Notes from a Path Less Travelled.

Introduction

I am a transplant surgeon who met Stephen and Linzi at the Salford Royal, Manchester on July 4, 2013. He was referred on to my team in the middle of May, 2013 for consideration of an intestinal transplant for a condition that was considered to be 'untreatable' by conventional techniques. Thus we started this incredible journey which culminated in me writing a few words to describe a special association that I was to share with this extraordinary man and his family in the coming months.

The Disease and Potential Cure

The call came from a colleague in Salford, Manchester, who we work closely with. It was a specific question as to whether we would consider someone for intestinal transplantation for a condition known as Pseudomyxoma Peritonei.

Intestinal transplantation in the UK had seen rejuvenation since two new centres; Oxford (for adults) and King's College London (for children) were designated for involvement in this highly specialised but low volume activity, in 2008. Before this event, two existing centres, Cambridge (for adults) and Birmingham (for children) contributed for the activity in the UK and it would be fair to say that not much had been achieved and the experience was limited. This is an important fact in Stephen's case since during subsequent discussions, it had come to light that Steve had in fact asked the question about an intestinal transplant, several years prior to me seeing him. I understand that his request was met with considerable negativity branding intestinal transplantation as an experimental procedure not worth exploring.

So the stage was set after this referral from a forward thinking physician at the Salford Royal Hospital, merely relaying a request from a patient who had just gone on to artificial feeding due to intermittent obstruction caused by the disease.

Pseudomyxoma Peritonei is a rare, benign tumour that mostly originates from the appendix and often, patients may have a history of appendicitis that required the appendix to be removed at a later date. This tumour is known for its production of a mucin-like material that coats the lining (peritoneum) of the abdomen as well as the intra-abdominal organs. It then causes a fibrous reaction and traps various anatomical parts of the intestine to cause pain and obstruction.

The conventional treatment for this condition revolves around the principle of stripping the peritoneal lining and 'de-bulking' as much of the disease attached to the bowel. This, in many cases, leads to the removal of the large bowel and a formation of a stoma. Furthermore, the peritoneal cavity is then treated with heated chemotherapy known has HIPEC therapy. This technique was described by Paul Sugarbaker and has been used extensively with good results. However, there are patients who may fail this therapy or may have disease that is not amenable to conventional therapy. These are the patients that we believe may benefit from an intestinal transplant and total reconstruction of their abdominal wall.

The Preparation

Since an intestinal transplant and total replacement of the abdominal wall for this disease had not been done before, careful planning at each step was crucial. The right questions needed to be asked and solutions sought and put in place before undertaking this operation. Firstly, Steve and Linzi were made aware of the fact that this was a path not explored by anybody in the past and therefore there was no guarantee that it would work. I had recently introduced the problem to a select group of intestinal transplant surgeons from all over the world at the biannual conference in Oxford.

The audience was divided in their opinion. This was reported back to Steve and Linzi who were undeterred by the international poll. Thus with this clear understanding that the procedure was a 'last ditch' effort in Steve's case to be rid of the tumour burden and restore the abdominal anatomy and physiology to as near normal as possible, we went ahead with the planning of such a manoeuvre.

The preparations were to be grouped in various stages. The process of evaluation for an intestinal transplant is essentially to answer three questions. Is it feasible? Is it safe? Is it going to be beneficial to the patient?

I needed to get more information about the biology of the tumour first hand. I was lucky to be able to contact and work with Tom Cecil, a surgeon and thinker extraordinaire, who had in fact taken care of Stephen when he was first diagnosed. My first contact with Tom was over the phone where I understandably got a mixed reaction of optimism and caution. Tom was very open to the fact that there may be another option for a small number of his patients that had failed conventional therapy and had progressed to intestinal failure.

We agreed to talk more over the course of the next week and he invited me over to his centre on a day that he had two cases booked for the Sugarbaker procedure. I duly attended that day in the operating room and understood the physical nature of the tumour during his operative session. This experience was invaluable to me and I couldn't thank Tom enough for that opportunity.

On returning from Tom's unit, I sent over Stephen's most recent CT scan to him for review at their multi-disciplinary meeting. It was thought that conventional surgery was truly not appropriate at that point. Also there were concerns of the tumour having 'invaded' the posterior aspect of the abdominal cavity through a muscle called the psoas.

What was reassuring though was the lack of tumour involvement in the substance of the liver or in the lungs. This was good news because it meant that the tumour was restricted to the abdominal cavity and had spared the liver. In addition the blood supply of the liver was patent and an extensive removal of all Stephen's stomach, duodenum, pancreas and small intestine was possible without compromising the blood supply of the liver.

Even though this fact was known, I wanted to cover all my bases and therefore invited a surgeon from Cambridge to come over and evaluate Stephen just in case we needed to either remove the liver en-bloc with the rest of the organs and then separate the liver from the tumour after cooling it down on the 'back-table', attach the new organs to the liver and then re-transplant the whole block in to Stephen (a process known as auto-transplantation of the liver). Unfortunately, this consult could not take place due to various reasons, but it turned out that such a manoeuvre was not required during the operation.

If there were a need to auto-transplant the liver, I would have needed a veno-venous bypass circuit that helps circulate the blood in Stephen's body by a machine. To facilitate this, I had a meeting with our cardiac surgeon who was very supportive and had agreed to help if such a manoeuvre was required. Thankfully, his expertise would not be needed as we managed to take the tumour out without the need for auto-transplanting the liver.

In addition to the modified multi-visceral graft (including the stomach, pancreas, duodenum and small intestine), Stephen was going to need replacement of his entire abdominal wall. The abdominal wall is a complex structure with different components including the skin, sub-cutaneous fat, muscle and a strong lining called the fascia. It keeps all the intra abdominal viscera in place. In Stephen's case this needed to be replaced because the tumour had encased it and had perforated through its layers at the site of his ileostomy. To enable this total replacement we make use of the abdominal wall from the same donor as the modified multivisceral graft. The plastic surgical team led by another gifted and extraordinary surgeon, Henk Giele, then transplants this. Henk and I developed the abdominal wall transplant programme in the UK and had done the first nine successful cases in the country. The concept of the abdominal wall transplant was not new. I had seen it first as a fellow with Dr Andreas Tzakis, my mentor, at the University of Miami where I had trained. However, Henk introduced a novel method of reconstituting the blood supply of this abdominal wall and is responsible for the success of the programme. I am in awe of his surgical expertise as well as his determination in achieving a 100 per cent result in his work. Henk had seen Stephen as part of his pre-transplant work-up and had gone through the procedure with him.

As the days went by during his pre-transplant evaluation, a few detrimental factors were beginning to emerge.

The tumour had managed to obstruct Stephen's stomach to an extent that he was 'drowning' in his own saliva. The saliva was regurgitating back up-wards through the oesophagus (food pipe) and entering his lungs. This is known as 'lung aspiration' and becomes the focus of an unrelenting lung infection.

In addition the tumour was causing obstruction to the ureters (tubes that carry urine from the kidney to the bladder). This required ureteric stents that were constantly getting infected from translocation of bugs from his obstructed bowel and was bringing Steve's overall condition down.

The tumour finally caused Stephen's bowel to rupture internally and cause an extensive abscess in his left sided psoas muscle. This made him very unwell indeed and needed a drain to be placed in an emergent situation.

Lastly, pressure from the tumour on Stephen's veins caused him to have an extensive clot in his left sided veins draining his leg, causing this leg to swell up and thus limiting movement.

In spite of these issues, Stephen was always on top form and would refuse to let these problems beat him. He was now limited to the hospital, but had an exercise bike in his room. He would bike between 5-15 kilometres a day depending upon how he was feeling.

After a protracted time of deliberation that included various tests on Steve's cardiac and respiratory status, psychological evaluation, nutritional, and general reserve, he was deemed suitable for the procedure at a local and national level and was put on to the transplant list.

The time one spends on the transplant wait list depends upon the blood group as well as an antibody profile that determines one's level of acceptance of another person's organs. It is known as the sensitization status of a patient. More sensitized patients wait a longer period for an organ. Stephen had no sensitization so was clear from that angle, however turned out to be a blood group B, a rare type for which he would have to wait for the right blood group. There was an option to use a universal donor blood group such as an O group that I wanted to be kept in reserve, in case he did not get an appropriate B group donor and time started running out in terms of Steve's physical status to withstand the operation.

Linzi

I have yet to come across a more involved, dedicated and strong person. Linzi has been the epitome of strength, equipoise, and inspiration especially at a very stressful time in both their lives. She had managed to define her role as a wife, partner and mother and distribute her energy and time in such a manner that none of the stakeholders felt left out. This is no easy feat considering the celebrity status and the limelight that a person like Stephen draws, as opposed to meeting the continued demands of energy and enthusiasm for the small things that a young family thrives on.

On one hand being on the frontline in Stephen's daily battle and then having the focus to engage with the children in their daily activities over the phone or the internet needed that special quality that Linzi definitely possesses. Her attitude towards Stephen's illness was selfless to say the least, always putting him and his incredible fight first.

T Minus 9 Days: Intensive Care

Stephen had an episode of acute onset of breathlessness. The tests showed that he possibly aspirated some of his saliva in to his lungs while asleep. He was immediately taken to the intensive care where efforts were made short of putting in a breathing tube down his trachea. These non-invasive methods of providing high pressure oxygen to patients entail wearing a head mask much like the ones seen on astronauts.

This was a big setback, because it was evident that the lung had taken a hit from the aspiration and could be the seat for infection.

The intensive care physician Dr Dyer was concerned that this may preclude him from getting a transplant. There was a palpable level of anxiety on both sides; physician and Stephen. Linzi was trying to put on a brave face for Stephen, but the writing was on the wall. He was requiring high doses of oxygen to keep the oxygen levels in his blood normal.

Then Stephen did what nobody expected. He recovered from this setback at a pace that shocked the intensivist. He was on a bike! Exercising! With the oxygen hood! Unbelievable! This was the level of his underlying physiology! No doubt to the testament of his life as a professional where he constantly challenged the status quo. He was out of the intensive care in a few days albeit supported by a small amount of oxygen breathed in through a nasal cannula. He was back and ready to take on the fight!

You can't imagine how much confidence this one episode gave me as a surgeon. All doubts about whether Steve would survive the operation vanished in a second. I knew he would come through it and I think he did too.

D-day

It started as a normal day. Stephen had had a few offers in the preceding days but they were not perfect and thus I had turned them down. There was a blood group B donor, whose family unfortunately declined consent for the bowel and abdominal wall.

Then came a perfect offer for Stephen, although it was a blood group O. The donor was in close vicinity of the transplant centre and made logistics easier. I went to see Stephen to talk to him about it. On my way in, I bumped in to Linzi who was making her way in to see him too. I told her about the offer, and it took a few seconds for her to register what I had just said. We both entered Stephen's room together.

Stephen had visitors and was in deep conversation with them before we interrupted and told him of the offer. It took him a few moments to register what he was told before he said, 'Bring it on, this is what I have been looking for'.

It is important to realise what he had been going through until that point.

Pain, from a perforated tumour on his skin, that would have been unbearable to any ordinary human was being tolerated by Steve only because of the hope that one day he will beat the cancer.

It was mind over matter. He was able to block out the pain, the restriction on his mobility, the restriction on his eating, drinking, tubes in his kidney, the urinary catheter, breathing difficulties, a tube in his back to drain the abscess created by the perforated bowel, the lack of a proper night's sleep; all in the hope that one day this offer of an organ would help him defeat the cancer that had destroyed his life. This was one driven man on a mission to get better.

As a surgeon, I couldn't have hoped for a better patient.

The Operation

Before the operation could take place, Stephen needed a device placed in his inferior vena cava that would trap any clots that attempted to break off from the major clot in his left leg. This was necessary to prevent what is known as pulmonary embolism where clots find their way in to the lungs and hamper appropriate oxygen exchange.

This inferior vena caval filter was placed by the interventional radiology consultant without much ado. Stephen had spent almost three months in the hospital and was known to majority of the hospital doctors.

I called Tom to let him know about the impending surgery. He was in London, having dinner with his mother on her birthday. He decided to take a taxi after dinner and make his way to the transplant centre to help with operation. It was midnight when we started. Such is this man's enthusiasm and determination.

The other teams were sounded. A cardiac anaesthesiologist, David Piggot, came in to help, in addition to the regular transplant team led by Peter Dimitrov. They got to work in placing the all-important lines for access to Stephen's circulation. There was a quiet air of anticipation since this was the first time such a procedure had been attempted. There were concerns about auto-transplantation of the liver and the need for the veno-venous bypass circuit. I confirmed with them in the initial team brief that according to the latest scans, I would not have to resort to that manoeuvre. I could see relief on Peter's face.

There are multiple teams involved in an intestinal transplant. There is a donor team that sets out to the donor hospital, evaluates, visualises the organs and gives the recipient team the green light to proceed if all looks good. The recipient team would ideally wait until such a signal is given, however, in Stephen's case the anticipated time required for removal of his tumour, bowel and abdominal wall was unknown and therefore we decided to start as early as possible. We knew from scans in the donor that the organs would be okay.

The plastic team was at hand to design the incision on Stephen's abdomen, because they would have to 'tailor' make it to the amount of tissue available from the donor. This again was different from all prior operations done together, because Stephen had tumour that had broken through his skin and needed total replacement of the abdominal wall.

The operation was carried out as a double act between me and Professor Peter Friend. Tom had made it in time to witness the start of the procedure. The approach was to go as wide as possible on the skin and explant his tumour and the encased non-functioning stomach, pancreas and intestine along with the abdominal wall. Care had to be taken to leave the blood supply of the liver intact. It is much like taking the whole engine out of a car along with its hood on its hinges without conventionally opening it for access to the engine.

Half-way through the procedure, we heard that the donor team were going to be delayed. There was a problem with a recipient of a heart from the same donor and therefore the cardiac team had to get in another recipient. This was a nightmare for us! Since we were making good progress in the resection of the tumour, we continued with our operation mindful of the fact that we may be done well before the organs arrived in the operating room. However, there was no other choice and we continued at our pace.

Finally, after careful operating, the tumour encasing the abdominal organs was removed leaving the liver in place with its normal arterial blood supply.

Now the liver derives its blood supply from two sources. One is the artery that we preserved and the other is the portal vein that shunts blood and nutrients from the intestine and delivers it to the liver for processing. In order to remove all Stephen's diseased intestine, it was imperative that we cut off this link and detach the intestine from the liver. In normal circumstances, if the new organs were ready for re-implantation, we would reconstitute the portal vein flow with the donor's vein. In Stephen's case there was a delay in the arrival of the organs, therefore we resorted to a well-described manoeuvre called a reno-portal anastomosis. Here one of Stephen's veins to the kidney is used as an inflow of blood via the portal vein in to the liver. This helps the liver maintain its nutrition till the new organs arrived.

The tumour was removed. The task was done! It was time to wait for the new organs. Stephen had managed to come through the process without as much as turning a hair. He was doing well on the operating table. The wait now was on for the arrival of his organs and it was time to take a break from operating. Tom and I met with Linzi outside the operating room and informed her of the progress made.

After an agonising wait, the organs arrived. They were appropriately prepared on the back table by Mr Reddy, consultant in-charge of the retrieval. And they were made ready for implantation. This went off without any problems and Stephen had a new set of 'insides'. It was an exhilarating moment to see the restoration of normal anatomy for this young man.

The appropriate connections were made and Stephen was handed over to Henk and his team that brought in the microscope to sew in the abdominal wall.

Usually, Henk and his team would temporarily sew the abdominal wall onto the patient's non-dominant forearm vessels whilst I was implanting the intestines. They would then transfer the abdominal wall graft on to the appropriate landing site once I was done and out of the way. However, in Stephen's case, since all the dissection to take out the tumour was already done, and we needed only 35 minutes to put the new organs in, Henk decided to wait and put the abdominal wall directly on to the intended landing site without using the forearm site. Steve, however, was aware of the fact that it may be sutured to his forearm and I believe it was one of the first things that he asked Linzi when he came around.

Henk and his team produced a beauty at the end and there was absolutely no evidence of the tumour inside or outside Stephen's body. He had won! He had defeated the cancer! Now he had to recover from the operation.

Tributes

Paul Sculthorpe MBE (Former Saints and Great Britain Captain and Challenge Companion)

I got to know Steve really well on the Paris to London Marathon challenge. There was only me and him, so we spent all our time together on that challenge and I realised what he was going through.

The stuff we did was tough for me but if you think of the condition Steve was in it was even more remarkable. After each day he was in bits to the point where he could not eat, and that gave me a real feel of what he was going through day to day.

To do the things he did in his condition was the mark of the man. That is why you could never say no to him on these challenges because every mile he asked someone to do, he was doing himself.

I have never met anybody so mentally tough who is willing to fight as much and push his own body as Steve. I turned my old phone on recently and I read through a text he sent me shortly before he passed away – and it said 'I'm feeling stronger and back on the bike' and this is just before his major transplant surgery. I just thought what a remarkable man.

People don't realise what he went through because he never told anybody. He was never one to feel sorry for himself and I suppose that is why he got to where he got to because he was positive. He was positive on making a recovery, positive in his outlook in trying to do good for other people.

It was devastating losing Steve but I am sure he will be so proud in what he has done. In the end, going for that ground breaking surgery and giving others a chance of following him is as big a legacy as anything he has done charity wise or sporting. He put his body on the line to try and save his own life but also to give other sufferers a chance as well.

He never knew when he was beaten and was like that as a player. I was fortunate to play with and against him and although never the biggest, he would always put his body on the line. Although he has such a remarkable story and was such an inspirational person, people should not forget that he was one of the top rugby league players.

The Race to the Grand Final – his last challenge and one that was too far for him – was tough. On that bike ride from Hull to Liverpool I've never been as close to throwing a towel in as I was that night because I was so drained going over Saddleworth Moor in the pouring rain. But then thought of Steve who was behind me and when you thought what he was going through I daren't even dream of packing in. Steve came in three-and-a-half hours behind our group and looked absolutely shot to pieces, but five hours later was first up to swim the River Mersey.

They tried to talk us out of swimming that day because the current was just so strong, but I just remember Precky, focused, determined and saying, 'Whatever he says I am swimming it, even if it is on my own.' He told people he was doing that and would not quit until he had swum the Mersey – as soon as Steve said that the rest of us followed and they let 10 of us do it.

He has a number of legacies – and I recall saying to Linzi not long after his death – that a lot of people can live for 90 years and won't achieve half of what Steve has done in 39 years he was here. We can look what he has packed into those 39 years and be thankful for it.

After being told the cancer would kill him, and being given months to live Steve always said he'd beat it and he did. It was the graft versus host that got him and that is so unfortunate, but he won his battle to be rid of cancer and it is important for people to know that because if Steve Prescott said he was going to do something he did it.

He was just a remarkable man and a lovely fella.

Dr Mark Saunders (Consultant Oncologist at The Christie)

Steve was an amazing man in so many ways. I first met him with Linzi back in 2007. He was recovering quickly from surgery and was apprehensive about starting chemotherapy.

Many patients receive chemotherapy and many cope well but others find it hard both physically and psychologically. However, Steve was not your 'typical' patient! He wanted to have treatment but also wanted to complete a series of 'challenges' for charity.

These challenges would be extreme for anybody, but to do them with this illness and with the effects of chemotherapy, well that takes real courage, determination and stamina. But these challenges motivated Steve and helped him push himself through chemotherapy.

I met him many times over this period until his tragic death. The whole aim of our treatment was to give him the best care available but also to fit this in with his family life and charity work.

I remember running with him with my son Charlie for a short arm of his five marathons challenge when he developed symptoms of bowel obstruction. Rather than stop and go to hospital, Steve just walked the last leg and carried on! I spoke to him then and he just didn't want to let anyone down. Typical of him.

I often spoke about Steve to other patients to try to motivate them at a very difficult time in their lives.

Steve was an inspirational man that treated his illness like another challenge and tried to beat it in the same way he beat opponents.

He will always be remembered and I do think he has left his mark on this world and his story will hopefully motivate other patients when they are faced with this awful illness. Linzi must be truly proud of her husband and his boys have a lot to live up to.

Tommy Martyn (Former Saints and Ireland Team-Mate, and Charity Walker)

I played with Steve first in the A team when I was coming back from injury. Steve was very dependable as a player; an extra pair of eyes in attack and defensively sound. A lot of the credit I got in the early years was down to him because he saw things and called them. If he told you to chip over he would get there. If I wanted him on my shoulder I knew he would be there because he was a man of his word.

If a bomb went up it was very rare that he dropped it and in attack he had pace to burn, as he showed playing for Hull when he out-paced Darren Albert.

A lot of kids get a knockback as teenagers and Steve was no exception, being told he was too small. He was always trying to lift heavy weights to counter that and put the size and bulk on. He had a determination to succeed that stood him in good stead and that was the making of him and something he carried to the end.

It was pleasing to take the double off Wigan in 1996 – a lot of us grew up together in first team rugby and we were a tight-knit group. When we won Super League we went out and partied hard, but we remained a tight bunch and that saw us through the first couple of years. It hurt Precky when he was told by the club he had to leave that team, and he always seemed to pick himself up for games against Saints.

When we heard the devastating news that he was terminally ill we did not know what to do. Eventually myself and Neil Holding phoned up Eric, his dad, and asked if we could see him. When we saw him he told us that he had no more tears to cry, that he had cried them all away.

It was upsetting to see our mate like that but after a few weeks you saw a tougher steel coming out of Steve Prescott.

I thought he would just roll over but he proved me wrong and faced it head on. That's the Steve Prescott we know and love, who always defied the odds and fought it through to the end.

Some of the challenges he did were mindblowing – getting off his sickbed to rise to the challenge even though he must have been suffering inside was utterly remarkable. Words can't describe how great a man he was.

What kept him going was to be the first person to get this multiple organ transplant and I'm glad he did. It is sad he is not here but he has pioneered something and hopefully long live his legacy.

He was so positive for someone who was ill. His message has got through to people that you can do it – you read things in the

Star now and people say they are doing this or that because of what Steve has done. Again that is a lasting legacy.

I was honoured to know Steve as a rugby league colleague, as a player, a good bloke but most importantly as a friend.

Martin Murray (World Middleweight Title Contender and First Pride of St Helens Winner)

I first got into rugby league as a schoolboy when Steve Prescott was in his pomp at Saints. He was just an awesome, talented player and was one of my heroes. You forget what an awesome rugby league player he was.

When he was diagnosed with cancer he went out and did all those challenges and had a never-say-die attitude. He would not let the cancer beat him.

The way he handled being terminally ill just proved what a special man he was. It is only at times like that you find out your true character – and what he showed and did after diagnosis was unbelievable.

The important thing now is to make sure his name lives on – and I am sure it will.

As an ambassador of the Steve Prescott Foundation I feel privileged and really appreciated. This is something close to my heart.

St Helens gets a lot of negativity but Steve was proud of his home town. By doing the Pride of St Helens Awards, and making a song and dance about how special the town really is, Steve has really put a positive message into people's mind about the borough and shown what talent we have got.

Despite Steve's own battles, he was selfless and considerate and supported me in my attempts to get a visa to get into America to box. I still have the absolutely lovely letter he wrote to support me. Given the position he was in, yet he was considerate about thinking of how he can help my career, it beggars belief. He did things like that for loads of people. What type of words can you find to pay tribute to a man like that. All you can think of is 'special' – he was special and you will be lucky if you ever meet another man like that, if ever.

Martin Blondel (Secretary Steve Prescott Foundation)

I was just a Saints fan and RL Fans website moderator who did not know Steve personally before he became ill – but we ended up being like brothers.

The first time I actually spoke to him was while helping organise the 1996 Legends game at Knowsley Road. It was not that long after his big operation at Basingstoke and Steve was only supposed to kick it off, but we could not get him off the field.

Out of everything we have done since the legends game is the pinnacle of what we have organised for the charity.

I got to know Steve well and he got stronger and more determined as time passed. He went from a person who was suffering from cancer to one who was so mentally strong and super human. The earliest sign of seeing that was on that first TransPennine walk when he showed the courage that made him stand out above anyone that I have ever met.

On the second walk he was different – both he and Tommy Martyn walked off ahead of the rest – and afterwards he said, 'I'll never do a walk again'. He wanted the tougher tests and throughout each and everyone he showed incredible resilience.

Steve and I came from different aspects of life. He was the sportsman while I was just an organiser from Royal Mail, who knew how to put an event on. I didn't know the sportsman's psyche, but he did not know how to organise events. We argued incessantly and then an hour later we would come back, usually with the right result. We had a special bond and Steve will always be my brother. I only knew him for seven years, but we spoke to each other twice a day. It was a fantastic partnership that we had.

Of all the fabulous experiences I have had in the Steve Prescott Foundation, and there have been many, travelling in the support boat to watch Steve, Chris Joynt, Bernard Dwyer, Ste Hall and Scully – five men with no rowing experience whatsoever – tackle the English Channel. Even though I broke my back on the speedboat coming back, it was so special to see how Steve and Scully got on with each other and how Scully protected Steve.

Steve leaves a lasting legacy – the SPF set up the St Helens 10K run and that started with 700 runners four years ago and we had

1,800 this year and could have taken more.

We also get inundated with letters from people with cancer, who tell us how Steve has inspired them not to give up. And the message that the fitter you can get yourself, the greater your chance of beating cancer was Steve's philosophy all the way through.

Steve wanted to show people there was an alternative to sitting on the couch, he wanted people to give themselves the best chance they had got of beating it. That is what Steve gave to people.

As a Foundation we will carry on inspiring people and supporting those facing adversity. It is not just those with cancer, people like Jimmy Gittins, Peter Stephenson and Paul Kilbride – all whose life changing injuries came from rugby.

It was the toughest time of my life when Steve died. I thought he had achieved the impossible by being cancer free. The amount of chats we had he made it clear that is all he ever wanted, no matter how slight a chance it was. But he got rid of it and when I got a phone call at 10pm which told me Steve's body had rejected his donor's anti-bodies and that it was crucial times I sat up all night and that was the first time that I thought we were no longer going to have him with us.

When I got the phone call in the morning, like everyone, I was numb and just went out and walked and walked, which Steve would have found funny.

Steve talks to me every day and still tells me off. We got to know each other so well that we both knew what the other was thinking and didn't have to say it.

Paul Wellens (St Helens Skipper and Former Great Britain Full Back)

Steve forced his way into the St Helens first team as I was a teenager watching from the terraces On the rugby field, despite not being big in stature you could tell he had a big heart and was a fierce competitor and that was one attribute I admired about him.

He was always very supportive of younger players and he was someone I looked up to when I was coming through the Saints junior system.

By the time I had made my way in the first team at St Helens,

Steve had moved on to Hull where he again gained huge admiration for the way he played the game.

That was evident when he ran the full length of the field against us in 2003 and 'There's only one Steve Prescott' rang around the KC Stadium. The try was that good I could have been forgiven for joining in with the opposition supporters.

The only time I got to play in the same game as Steve was for Lancashire v Yorkshire in what was to be the last match of his career after picking up a serious knee injury from which he couldn't recover. Despite it being very brief at least I got the opportunity to line up in the same side as Steve, something I'm very grateful for.

Since then our paths crossed more frequently as our children attend the same school and occasionally we would talk about sporting topics but rugby league in particular.

I remember arriving home from training one day and hearing the news that Steve had been diagnosed with a rare form of cancer, it obviously came as a huge shock and I remember thinking how Steve would respond but never in my wildest dreams did I imagine a response like the one we got.

Not only did Steve tackle the disease head on but he has brought so much good out of what was a very difficult and emotional situation.

Obviously he has raised huge amounts of money by taking on challenges that quite frankly seem crazy and he has really pulled the community together, both the Rugby League community and especially the community in our home town of St Helens.

His selfless attitude was quite staggering and despite the struggles he faced on a daily basis he seemed to be always asking and caring about the wellbeing of others. The phrases 'legend' and 'role model' get used quite often but for me Steve goes to the top of the list in both categories.

And more than anything he was a devoted family man, his wife Linzi is lovely and they have two fantastic children, if we're proud of Steve and his achievements then I could only imagine how proud those closest to him are.

I'm privileged to be able to call him a friend because there really is 'Only one Steve Prescott.' And we will never forget that.

Neil Prescott (Steve's Brother)

I used to think cancer is a thing that won't happen to me or my family. Then when it does happen you seem to wake up to the fact that it is in everyday life. Every day people are affected somehow, maybe we are blind to the fact that it is everywhere.

When Ste phoned me that Friday, I'd had a feeling for weeks something wasn't right but I shut it out thinking all was okay. It was like a part of me had been ripped apart, how could this happen to my younger brother. My world fell apart.

I just didn't care about things anymore, my views on life changed and I began to take on a different perspective to the ways I'd known.

But seeing Ste take on a different route to the one he was used to made me realise that people really do need to live life to the full and I hope he keeps being an inspiration to all people. (I'm proud to be his older brother).

Ste always said people who are sick should not just sit back and give up but embrace life to the full, everyone has a purpose in life.

God bless you Ste.

Shaun McRae (Former Head Coach at St Helens and Hull FC)

I first met Steve Prescott in January 1996 when I began my tenure as Head Coach with St Helens. He made an immediate impact displaying commitment and dedication that you would expect of a professional athlete.

The one thing I realised very quickly is that I didn't need to search for a fullback. I didn't know then, but I would learn later on in Steve's career that I had been privileged to coach one of the best fullbacks that the British game had ever produced.

When you coach players, it's not just about on the field, you need a relationship, albeit doesn't mean you have to become best friends. There has to be a distance, yet mutual respect if you're going to work together and get the best out of each other. Steve and I had a great working relationship, I believe we challenged each other all the time. He constantly sought feedback on performances, he was always asking questions and seeking ways to improve whether it be skill based, positional play, size and strength, Steve didn't mind, he just had to be the best he could possibly be.

When Steve made a decision to leave St Helens and sign at Hull FC, I never thought our paths would cross again as player/coach. The year was 2001, Steve had really developed his game. He had now played over 180 Super League games, yet he still wasn't satisfied with his game. Steve sought perfection, he desired success, he valued excellence, and he appreciated his team mates and was never going to let them nor himself down.

When I learnt of Steve's illness in 2006, and the reports of his life expectancy, I couldn't stop my thoughts being transported to the days of Knowsley Road and the Boulevard and seeing Steve Prescott fight to lift heavier in the gym, compete in all the conditioning sessions, contest every drill like he had to win and fight for every metre gained on the field. With that wisdom, I knew Steve would use the same processes to fight for himself and his wonderful family and friends.

Steve's desire and positive outlook has been and will always be an inspiration to us all. He never blamed anyone, he never asked anyone to do something he couldn't, he never backed down. He strove to help others, he kept himself involved with the game that he loved so much and yet was entitled to be dismissive.

I mentioned earlier about coaches and players not having to become best friends, Steve and I didn't, but our friendship was much closer and open after I finished coaching him. That is why I am so honoured to be contributing to this book.

To have known Steve Prescott was a pleasure, to have worked with Steve Prescott was a privilege, to see the effect Steve Prescott has had on other people is amazing.

Steve was a credit to the great game of Rugby League, a credit to his wonderful family and a credit to himself.

Perhaps it is all best summed up by the title 'Steve Prescott Man of Steel Award.'

Steve McNamara (England Coach, Former Hull and Wakefield Team-Mate)

Superhuman – that's one of the best ways to describe Steve Prescott.

His physical and mental feats in dealing with not only his illness but the challenges he took on are way beyond what a human should be able to do.

The last years of Stephen's life since the diagnosis of his cancer means he will always be remembered for those feats and rightly so, but what we also need to remember him as was the brilliant free flowing natural rugby league player that brought great joy to everyone that witnessed him play. His ability to do things that others said he couldn't stemmed from being told he was too small to play at the highest level – he proved them wrong and continued to prove people wrong throughout his life.

It is a lesson for us all. Way above all of that though for me was Stephen's qualities as a husband, a father, a son, a brother and a friend to many.

With so much of Stephen's life being shared out in public the private side of it is something that many won't know. I had the fortune to travel with Stephen from Hull to Wakefield on a daily basis when we played for the Wildcats – I got to know him closely and the love for his family and friends was clearly evident.

We enjoyed many a lively debate on various aspects of life, he always had an opinion and was never shy of expressing it. I learnt a lot from him and will always be grateful for the time we got to spend together and the positive impact he made on me personally.

Stephen was and will continue to be an inspiration to us all.

God bless you mate.

Kris Radlinski (Former Wigan, England and Great Britain Full Back, Rugby General Manager, Wigan Warriors)

They say that you never forget where you were when significant moments take place in your life. I was just pulling into Twickenham railway station – I was there to watch Joel Tomkins make his England RU debut – when I received a text from my sister, telling me Steve Prescott had sadly passed away. A tear ran down my face as the realisation that Steve's fight was over.

But what a fight it was.

Having played against Steve for most of my career, we forged a friendship built on respect. The fullbacks union always stuck together, and even though we played for opposing teams in the sport's greatest contest – the Wigan-St Helens derbies – we always found time to show appreciation.

Steve was quite the showman on the field. He usually scored a try with flair; always with a smile on his face.

To become an accomplished full back you need a mixed skill-set, with 'bravery' high up on the list. But the bravery he exuded on the rugby field was nothing compared to what he displayed once he was diagnosed with terminal cancer.

Most people sink into their shell when greeted with such news – and stay there.

Steve was the opposite.

His heart must have been ripped to shreds by the news. But then, incredibly, he gained strength from it. He was a hero to his loving wife and their two sons, and vowed to fight the illness with everything he had.

His bravery inspired others. Along his journey, he gathered an impressive group of people – including many old team-mates and opponents – who dedicated their lives to his great fight.

The fund-raising challenges they undertook were extreme for fit, healthy athletes: multi-marathons, climbing mountains, cycling the length and breadth of countries. They covered hundreds of miles, raising thousands of pounds.

For Steve, weakened by both the illness which had invaded his body and the drugs which helped control it, those challenges were amplified. They became monumental, seemingly impossible tasks.

But still he carried on, pedalling, walking, running and most of all fighting.

And he did it all without a shred of self-pity. That's what struck me the most about Steve – the way he lived with such great humility. Not once did he crave sympathy or hanker for attention.

When I saw him, he always asked how I was and how my family was. He took interest in what I was doing in my life.

He faced challenges that I couldn't begin to imagine but he made time to ask about me. He wasn't preoccupied with his own battle, he wanted to help others with theirs – no matter how small in comparison.

Ultimately, the way he lived his life shaped the legacy following his death.

He has left us with many memories and a foundation which will continue to help others. The renaming of the Man of Steel in his honour ensures his name will live on in the sport he loved.

But more than that, he showed us all that we must face adversity with the ultimate passion, and taught us that great things are often achieved when things can't get any worse. That is what made Steve such a great man.

I feel lucky and proud that rugby league has given me so many highlights. And when I learned Steve had asked me to write this tribute, I was both humbled and honoured – even if words, however lavish, seem almost limiting in describing Steve Prescott.

And that's coming from a Wiganer, to a guy from St Helens.

Mike Denning (Chairman, Steve Prescott Foundation)

I will never forget the day I was present with Steve's close friends when we received the call from Steve himself to say he had been diagnosed with a rare form of cancer and that he had been told that there was no realistic chance of survival. Eccleston Park Golf Club was the venue and I had just taken another thrashing at golf.

Time stood still. Nobody could take in the news and frantic calls were made to try and establish if the story, even though it had come from Ste himself, was correct. To say we were all in shock is an understatement. A friend, one of the lads, fit sportsman, this couldn't be correct. Little did I know or appreciate that the day would change my life forever.

I had known Ste through some of his mutual friends Paul Barrow and Mike Ford. I had stood on the terraces to witness Steve's bravery as a somewhat diminutive figure holding his own in the full back role at Saints and then at Hull. We had shared some fun nights together and he was just a regular guy who liked a laugh and could be full of mischief. He was always a professional and had a massive will to win.

Steve's career is set out in the book but having been asked to get involved in his fund raising activities I became close to Ste and his family and shared some of his highs and lows during his battle against pseudomyxoma peritonei.

In every challenge Steve became involved in he showed a spirit and determination to succeed that I have never seen in another individual. He made it look that the disease which was constantly aggravating him was a mere irritation. As the medics will tell you there is no answer other than his total mental toughness that allowed him to achieve his goals. I am still in awe of this super human effort. Like us all he had his faults and he could complain and moan like the best of us but what Steve Prescott had in my view could never be replicated.

An MBE for Steve was more than well deserved but there is nothing that could have rewarded him for his bravery other than the gift of life itself. It is an old cliché but the good and the young die far too early but for those who knew Steve Prescott MBE he has left us enriched and better people for his friendship.

The world has lost a great man and I have lost a dear friend from whom I have learnt a lot. He battled and won his final fight only to be taken in unforeseen circumstances. I am privileged the Foundation in his name as Chairman and will be grateful more than he will ever know for his friendship and lessons he taught us all.

He will never be forgotten and his time with us meant so much. I know he will always look over us all and rests well now his work is done.

Tom Cecil (Consultant Surgeon, Basingstoke and North Hampshire Hospital)

I first met Steve in October 2006. It was a devastating time for him and Linzi having been diagnosed with advanced pseudomyxoma cancer with their young child Taylor and recently newborn baby Koby.

He was facing the daunting prospect of a huge operation with no guarantee of success.

We operated in November 2006 and removed 80 per cent of Steve's tumour but having to remove his whole colon giving him a permanent stoma bag on the stomach, something he dreaded as a young man and professional sportsman.

He bounced back from this and with his iron will and love and support from Linzi set about rebuilding his life. He went on to achieve feats that I and many would not have thought possible running marathons, rowing the English Channel and always on a hectic schedule busy and fundraising.

Unfortunately Steve's cancer progressed, blocking his bowel and with conventional surgery no longer an option he explored the possibility of small bowel transplantation which had never been performed for this condition before.

Meeting and talking to Steve and Linzi was a privilege and their humour and generosity of spirit for those of us involved and others who may benefit with the disease, inspired and led us to move ahead. I was touched by his calm and noble approach and the feeling of being in the presence of greatness that those who spent time with Steve will understand.

Tragically Steve whilst getting through the operation later died from complications. It was a privilege to know and treat Steve and his bravery and vision has opened up a new field that will be explored and one day offer the hope and future to others that epitomised Steve Prescott.

Chris Joynt (Former St Helens Captain and Ireland Team-Mate)

When Steve first came into the Saints set-up he was not the biggest of guys, but over time he overcame that by training the house down and becoming physically strong enough to hold a place down.

After being written off as being too small he went on to play for his beloved Saints – and that is all he wanted.

What people underestimated with Precky was his lightning pace and he could certainly exploit a gap and there are times that you need to be like a whippet.

Precky was part of that young team coming through in 1996 and we hadn't seen the best of it in that double-winning year.

Nobody ever wants to leave the Saints, but circumstances meant Steve was sold to Hull at the end of 1997. In subsequent matches he always raised his game against Saints, going the full length to beat Darren Albert in 2003 and even skinning us a couple of times when he played at Wakefield.

I played alongside him for Ireland in the 2000 World Cup and although we were the underdogs, we had a side packed with quality players. We could turn it on when required and we won all of our group games.

What Steve did after being diagnosed with cancer was amazing. He never looked ill and I used to joke with him about that when he was running another marathon or at the front of another challenge on his bike. However, deep down every day was such a fight for him – he was simply putting on a brave face.

With regards to the challenges, I was with Steve's five-man crew that rowed the English Channel which was one of the hardest things we did. The beauty of that was that Steve simply picked up the phone the night before and 12 hours later three lads had joined him in rowing the Channel – but that was the pull he had.

None of us had never been in a rowing boat, let alone rowed across the busiest shipping lane in Europe. We had some tough hours in that boat, but to get to the other side and see everyone's faces was amazing and even we thought 'How did we do that?'

Steve was like a Sport Billy – he could play anything – rugby, golf, football, he could do anything. He was a good all rounder and very knowledgeable about sport too.

What Steve did while he was alive has left a legacy, but for it to continue he needs a lot of support. It is important for everybody else to do their bit.

People forget that behind every good man there is a good woman and his wife Linzi is testament to that. She knew him better than any of us and must miss him so much every day, but the way she has conducted herself and is bringing the boys up is great to see.

It will be wonderful in years to come if his two lads can row the Channel or run the London Marathon – and that really would keep the Steve Prescott name alive.

George Riley (BBC Sports Presenter)

I got to know Steve, like many others, through his charity work.

I will always feel extremely fortunate that I had the opportunity to experience both his friendship and his extraordinary selflessness in the face of the most painful adversity imaginable.

Steve was a brilliant rugby league player. This is often forgotten because of the legendary fundraising legacy he has left. On the pitch he was as respected as he was off it.

We became close friends in the final few years of his life.

One powerful memory was sharing a touchline hug at Old Trafford before the 2012 Grand Final. I was broadcasting, Steve delivering the matchball from his final charity challenge. We stood chatting as he waited to be introduced to 70,000 fans, his trademark air of embarrassment that so many people would actually care about him. Steve told me then he was done. Mentally and physically. He could take no more. But still he fought on for one more year.

The last time I saw Steve was at his home, just before being taken down to Oxford for the surgery we hoped would give him a new start. His wonderful sons were playing football in the garden as Taylor waited for his granddad to take him to training with Liverpool FC. Faced with life or death surgery, Steve's main concern was to apologise for making me drive to see him because he wasn't well enough to travel. He was always apologising for having his mates visit in hospital saying, 'I know hospitals are horrible places to visit'. Of course he knew.

When Steve entered his final chapter, we were chatting about running the London Marathon together. Deep down I feared I'd be running it alone but Steve still hoped that if he could survive 2013 then the next year would be better.

He was a great laugh – the boxing booze up with Scully, Jimmy and the boys was memorable, a loyal friend – it was always about what he could do for you and not vice versa, and a brilliant bloke.

I'm gutted to have lost Steve and think about him every day. But I'm happy that in those extra seven years that he fought to live, Steve got the chance to be a great dad, husband and mate, and show the world what a legend he was.

Whatever I do with the rest of my life I will forever strive to be more like Steve.

Miss you mate.

John Prescott (Former Deputy Prime Mininster)

Steve Prescott was a wonderful adopted son of Hull. Although I never met him, I greatly admired him so was surprised and delighted when he asked me to write a tribute.

One question hangs in the air from our shared surname. My father was from St Helens before he moved to Liverpool, so I may have had family there. It is a shame I never got the chance to ask him if we could have been related – I would like to think somewhere we were because if you wanted to be related to someone it would be a man like Steve Prescott.

Steve was an idol and hero in Hull, which was as much to do with his character in dealing with that terrible illness as it was to do with his rugby.

What made Steve so extraordinary was his positivity. You hear stories of inspirational people, but when you see them do what they do when you know what must be in their minds you cannot help but admire them. He had a real desire to make a difference with whatever time he had, and despite all those difficulties and adversities he endured he certainly did that, showing great tenacity and community spirit. No wonder he has earned such admiration.

Steve's personality came across in his actions – he was not a self centred person or bothered about promoting himself. He thought of others and you can't have a greater credit than that. Although I did not know him personally, I knew that much about him – and so did the people of Hull who took him to their hearts.

Hull is really a big village with a big heart – and one with great loyalties and friendship. And Steve was really admired as an adopted son of the city. Although he was a Hull FC player he had a capacity to unite the rugby followers across the city, black and white and red and white, when he undertook his challenges.

Steve's legacy is the recognition of the courage of a man who worked for others when his time was limited, doing it with a smile on his face. It was not that he just appealed for some funds, he got out and did it.

When people read about Steve Prescott they see an amazing story from an amazing man.

Steve Crooks (Former Hull Coach)

I was up at Hull's training ground in September, 2006 when Linzi phoned and told me the awful news about Steve's diagnosis. She was in floods of tears when she said, 'Crooksy – it's Steve, they have said he's dying.'

Immediately I shot around to their house and Linzi opened the door with new-born Koby in her arms. She explained that Steve was upstairs and wouldn't come down.

I asked to go up, and ridiculously I walked into his bedroom and on seeing Steve in a heap on the bed said, 'Now then Precky, how are you?' It just came out and he responded with a few expletives and said that he was gone. But the biggest thing that will stick in my mind was his comment that he would not see his kids grow up.

I didn't know what I was going to say – we were both upset and then I said, 'Why don't you curl up in the corner and die then, despite the fact you have a brand new baby downstairs. Linzi has just opened the door with your son in her arms.'

'If you are going to die, then let's have a battle.'

I had just read Lance Armstrong's books and, although he is disgraced now, he had made a science out of investigating what was wrong with him and wouldn't take no for an answer. That was my inspiration when I said to Steve, 'I don't care what the nurse said, but if you are going to die then at least let's have a fight. If you don't want to do it for yourself, do it for the boys and Linzi.'

We were up there a couple of hours and the talk perked him up a bit and basically the end result was that we went downstairs to Linzi, his mum and dad and Koby. It was time for him to start his battle. There were no heroics in that from me, it was just a bit of inspiration that I'd got from the books.

Steve was on the starting line – and we had started with a reason to fight.

Precky was a great player but his problem – and one we'd joke about it in the dressing room – was that he was worrier. If there was an announcement on Beijing flu coming in that evening, then he would have contracted it the night before.

Even in warm up before a game he'd say, 'I have got a pull here and an ache there', but once you got him out on the field it wasn't a problem – he just played. So bearing in mind someone with that attitude went on to deal with what he did was quite remarkable. The fight that came out of him in those last seven years was incredible and inspirational that is why he survived for so long.

And in that battle the people responded to him, not simply because of his fight against cancer, but due to the type of person he was, inspirational. Precky was a lovely bloke, one who didn't have a bad word for anybody. He was the fella you wanted in your team, on your night out or at your family do. You wanted him to be with you with whatever you were doing because he was such a good lad.

At Hull Sharks, when he first joined from Saints, it was adversity from day one, but we tried to make a fist of it. Precky was thrown into an environment that wasn't conducive to performing to the best of your ability, and a difficult time for all involved within the club at that time. But he came here and embraced it. He took Hull to his heart and equally the fans responded. After leaving Hull and having a spell at Wakefield, the fans here were really delighted and loved it when Precky returned because they realised what a great player and decent bloke he was.

They saw his qualities as a player – he was deceivingly quick and scored some great tries for the club where he showed how fleet of foot and how very aware he was.

Although Steve will always be regarded as a St Helens bloke Hull have claimed a piece of him because of who he was and what he did. They have an even bigger piece of him now given what went on afterwards with his fight against cancer. Hull is a tough place and they don't take people to heart without justification, but the city loved him.

The typical thing about Precky was his care for everyone else and that was reflected greatly in his challenges, which were all aimed at what he could do for other people. He cared and that was massively important in the impact he had on me.

With Steve it was always about others and not himself and that is testament to the man that shall live with us forever and a day.

Statistics

Stephen Prescott – Club Record

St Helens RLFC

Season	Apps	Tries	Goals	DG	Points
1993-94	13+2	3	29	0	70
1994-95	34	20	5	0	90
1995-96	21	8	15	0	62
1996	27	15	17	0	94
1997	20	6	0	0	24
Total	115+2	52	66	0	340

Debut v Leigh (H) SBC 19/09/93 (Sub)
Last match v Penrith Panthers (A) WCC 25/07/97
Honours – Challenge Cup Winners 1996 1997; Super League Champions 1996

Hull Sharks (First Spell)

Season	Apps	Tries	Goals	DG	Points
1998	21	8	20	0	72
1999	19	7	43	2	116
Total	40	15	63	2	188

Debut v Whitehaven (A) CC 15/02/1998
Last match v Sheffield Eagles (H) SL 12/09/99

Statistics

Stephen Prescott – Club Record

St Helens RLFC

Season	Apps	Tries	Goals	DG	Points
1993-94	13+2	3	29	0	70
1994-95	34	20	5	0	90
1995-96	21	8	15	0	62
1996	27	15	17	0	94
1997	20	6	0	0	24
Total	115+2	52	66	0	340

Debut v Leigh (H) SBC 19/09/93 (Sub)
Last match v Penrith Panthers (A) WCC 25/07/97
Honours – Challenge Cup Winners 1996 1997; Super League Champions 1996

Hull Sharks (First Spell)

Season	Apps	Tries	Goals	DG	Points
1998	21	8	20	0	72
1999	19	7	43	2	116
Total	40	15	63	2	188

Debut v Whitehaven (A) CC 15/02/1998
Last match v Sheffield Eagles (H) SL 12/09/99

Wakefield Trinity Wildcats

Season	Apps	Tries	Goals	DG	Points
2000	24+1	3	13	0	38

Debut v Leigh (A) CC 13/02/00
Last match v London Broncos (H) SL 20/08/00

Hull FC (Second Spell)

Season	Apps	Tries	Goals	DG	Points
2001	26	17	55	1	179
2002	22	6	7	0	38
2003	19	18	72	0	216
Total	67	41	134	1	433

Debut v Keighley CC 11/02/2001
Last match v Wakefield Trinity Wildcats (H) SL 26/06/03

Stephen Prescott – Representative Record

Season	Team	Apps	Tries	Goals	DG	Points
1994-95	GB U21s	2	1	3	0	10
1996	England	2	3	7	0	26
2000 (WC)	Ireland	4	1	17	0	38
2003	Lancs	1	0	0	0	0